HANDBOOK OF
Critical Care Nursing

HANDBOOK OF
Critical Care Nursing

Carolyn M. Hudak, PhD, RN
Nurse Practitioner
Denver, Colorado

Barbara M. Gallo, RN, MS, CNAA
Assistant Professor
University of Hartford
School of Education,
   Nursing and Health Professions
Division of Nursing
Hartford, Connecticut

J.B. Lippincott Company
Philadelphia

Sponsoring Editor: Diana Intenzo
Project Editor: Amy P. Jirsa
Indexer: Alberta Morrison
Design Coordinator: Melissa G. Olson
Interior Designer: Anne O'Donnell
Cover Designer: Tom Jackson
Production Manager: Helen Ewan
Production Coordinator: Kathryn Rule
Compositor: Circle Graphics
Printer/Binder: R. R. Donnelley & Sons Co./Crawfordsville
Cover Printer: New England Book Components, Inc.

6 5 4 3 2 1

Library of Congress Cataloging-in-Publication Data

Hudak, Carolyn M.
    Handbook of critical care nursing / Carolyn M. Hudak, Barbara M.
Gallo.
        p. cm.
    Includes index.
    ISBN 0-397-55026-X
    1. Intensive care nursing—Handbooks, manuals, etc. I. Gallo,
Barbara M. II. Title.
    [DNLM: 1. Critical Care—nurses' instruction. WY 154 H883h 1994]
RT120.I5H82 1994
610.73'61—dc20
DNLM/DLC
for Library of Congress   93-21270
                                                                  CIP

Any procedure or practice described in this book should be applied by the healthcare practitioner under appropriate supervision in accordance with professional standards of care used
with regard to the unique circumstances that apply in each practice situation. Care has been
taken to confirm the accuracy of information presented and to describe generally accepted
practices. However, the authors, editors, and publisher cannot accept any responsibility for
errors or omissions or for any consequences from application of the information in this book
and make no warranty express or implied, with respect to the contents of the book.

Every effort has been made to ensure drug selections and dosages are in accordance with
current recommendations and practice. Because of ongoing research, changes in government
regulations and the constant flow of information on drug therapy, reactions and interactions,
the reader is cautioned to check the package insert for each drug for indications, dosages,
warnings and precautions, particularly if the drug is new or infrequently used.

CONTENTS

Ventilators

COPD and ARDS

Pulmonary Drugs

5 The Renal System   99

Assessment and Diagnosis

Acute Renal Failure

Nervous System

Gastrointestinal System

Endocrine System

Multisystem Conditions

Appendix—ACLS Guidelines for Non–Life-Threatening Situations   349

HANDBOOK OF
Critical Care Nursing

CHAPTER 1
Legal Issues

Jurisdictions That Have Living Will Statutes*

Alabama	Kansas	Ohio
Alaska	Kentucky	Oklahoma
Arizona	Louisiana	Oregon
Arkansas	Maine	Rhode Island
California	Maryland	South Carolina
Colorado	Minnesota	South Dakota
Connecticut	Mississippi	Tennessee
Delaware	Missouri	Texas
District of Columbia	Montana	Utah
Florida	Nevada	Vermont
Georgia	New Hampshire	Virginia
Hawaii	New Jersey	Washington
Idaho	New Mexico	West Virginia
Illinois	North Carolina	Wisconsin
Indiana	North Dakota	Wyoming
Iowa		

*As of November, 1991. To update this information, contact Concern for Dying at (212) 246-6973.

Jurisdictions Authorizing Health Care Proxy/Agent Appointments*

Arkansas	Nevada
Connecticut	New Jersey
Delaware	New York
District of Columbia	South Carolina
Florida	Texas
Idaho	Utah
Massachusetts	Virginia
Minnesota	Wyoming
Montana	

*As of November 11, 1991.

CHAPTER 2
The Elderly Patient

Developmental Tasks of the Elderly

Decision of where and how to live for their remaining years

Preservation of supportive, intimate, and satisfying relationships with spouse, family, and friends

Maintenance of adequate and satisfying home environment relative to health and economic status

Provision of sufficient income

Maintenance of maximum level of health

Attainment of comprehensive health and dental care

Maintenance of personal hygiene

Maintenance of communication and adequate contact with family and friends

Maintenance of social, civic, and political involvement

Initiation of new interests (in addition to former activities) that increase status

Recognition and feeling of being needed

Discovery of meaning in life after retirement and when confronted with illness of self/spouse and death of spouse and other loved ones; adjustment to death of loved ones

Development of a significant philosophy of life, and discovery of comfort in a philosophy/religion

Nursing Interventions for Hearing Impaired Patients

Stand close and face patient.

Touch patient to get attention before communicating (personal space should be protected).

Speak slightly louder and slowly. (Do not shout.)

Pause more often than usual.

Avoid exaggerated lip movement.

Use facial expressions and gestures.

Use short phrases.

Repeat misinterpreted communication using different words.

Don't turn and walk away while talking.

Help family/support system with communication techniques.

Discourage social withdrawal (a problem associated with hearing loss).

Make sure hearing device works properly.

Nursing Interventions for Visually Impaired Patients

Identify yourself on approach.

Approach blind patients from the front.

Assess impact of failing vision and patient's ability to adapt both during hospitalization and after discharge.

Instill all prescribed medications.

Assess stress level because increased stress can necessitate higher dosages of eye medication for patients with glaucoma.

Be alert to side effects that other medications may have on the eyes (ie, medications containing antihistamines, caffeine, and atropinelike substances).

Provide eye lubrications when eyes are dry.

Symptoms of Acute Confusion

Disorders of Cognition

Impairment in perception, memory, and thinking

Behavior includes
 disorientation for location and time
 confusion of unknown persons with familiar ones
 memory impairment
 delusions that food is poisoned

Abnormal Sleep–Wake Cycle

Disorders of attention, vigilance, and sleep dysfunction

Behavior includes
 insomnia
 vivid night dreams
 agitation as darkness occurs ("sundown syndrome")
 reduced attention time
 under-alertness or over-alertness
 fluctuating awareness from drowsiness to lucidity

Disorders of Psychomotor Behavior

Generally nonspecific

Behavior includes
 wandering
 fluctuation from intense agitation to somnolence
 combative behavior, usually due to fear

Possible Reversible Causes of Acute Confusion

Pharmacological factors:	Narcotics, sedatives, digitalis, tranquilizers, steroids, antihypertensives, antidepressants, diuretics, chemotherapeutic agents, bronchodilators, anticholinergics
Environmental factors:	Abrupt change in environment, sensory deprivation, sensory overload, isolation
Psychosocial factors:	Depression, loss, grief
Nutritional imbalances:	Vitamin deficiencies (B_{12}, folic acid, niacin), starvation
Elimination imbalances:	Fecal impaction, urinary retention
Trauma:	Fractures, surgery, concussion/contusion, subdural hematoma, cerebral hemorrhage
Alcohol abuse:	Alcohol withdrawal when hospitalized may be overlooked
Pain:	Due to trauma of external or internal origin
Fluid and/or electrolyte imbalances:	Sodium excess of depletion, dehydration, acid–base imbalance
Metabolic factors:	Hypo- or hyperthyroidism, renal impairment, liver malfunction
Cardiovascular factors:	Congestive heart failure, hypotension, myocardial infarction, dysrhythmias
Bacteriological factors:	Infection (eg, pneumonia)
Body temperature:	Hyperthermia, hypothermia

Summary of Cognitive Changes With Aging

Intelligence

Remains stable

More hesitant with new tasks

Learning

Takes longer to respond

Needs motivation to learn new material

Memory

Decline in short-term memory

Remote memory remains intact

CHAPTER 3
The Cardiovascular System

Suggested Monitoring Lead Selection

Lead	Rationale for Use
II	• Produces large, well formed P waves and QRS complexes for strip interpretation
	• Produces large ECG signal for easy monitoring
MCL₁	• Produces characteristic BBB configuration for differentiating RBBB from LBBB, VEA from aberrancy, and RV from LV ectopy
	• Produces well formed P waves for analyzing atrial dysrhythmias
III, AVF, Lewis Lead (& II, MCL₁)	• Produce well formed P waves, helpful in identifying atrial dysrhythmias
I	• Use with patients in respiratory distress to decrease motion artifact; affected less by chest movement than other leads

ECG, electrocardiogram; BBB, bundle branch block; R(L)BBB, right (left) bundle branch block; VEA, ventricular ectopic activity; RV, right ventricle; LV, left ventricle.

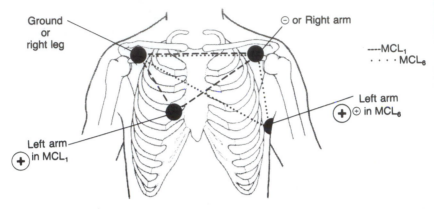

System for obtaining simulation of V_1 and V_6 chest leads. For an MCL tracing, use lead "I" selection.

Advantages and Disadvantages of Bipolar and Unipolar Lead Systems

	Unipolar	Bipolar
Distance between electrical poles	30–50 cm	1–3 cm
Sensitivity	More sensitive to intracardiac electrical activity (may sense depolarization from a different chamber)	Less sensitive to intracardiac/extracardiac electrical activity (less likely to oversense)
	More sensitive to extracardiac electrical activity (may sense myopotentials)	
Muscle twitching	May occur due to electric signals picked up near the pulse generator	Rare occurrence because both electrodes are intracardiac
Pacemaker artifact	Large; may distort QRS complex	Small; less distortion of QRS complex
Insertion	Easier to place	More difficult to place
Uses	Bipolar systems can be converted to unipolar if needed	Temporary/permanent systems
		Must be used in conjunction with the internal cardiovertor–defibrillator

Electrocardiogram (ECG) Monitor Problem Solving

Excessive Triggering of Heart Rate Alarms

- Is high-low alarm set too close to patient's rate?
- Is monitor sensitivity level set too high or too low?
- Is patient cable securely inserted into monitor receptacle?
- Are the lead wires or connections damaged?
- Has the monitoring lead been properly selected?
- Were the electrodes applied properly?
- Are the R and T waves the same height, causing both waveforms to be sensed?
- Is the baseline unstable, or is there excessive cable or lead wire movement?

Baseline But No ECG Trace

- Is the size (gain or sensitivity) control properly adjusted?
- Is appropriate lead selector being used on monitor?
- Is the patient cable fully inserted into ECG receptacle?
- Are electrode wires fully inserted into patient cable?
- Are electrode wires firmly attached to electrodes?
- Are electrode wires damaged?
- Is the patient cable damaged?
- Call for service if trace is still absent.
- Is the battery dead (for telemetry system)?

Intermittent Trace

- Is patient cable fully inserted into monitor receptacle?
- Are electrode wires fully inserted into patient cable?
- Are electrode wires firmly attached to electrodes?
- Are electrode wire connectors loose or worn?

Intermittent Trace (continued)

- Have electrodes been applied properly?
- Are electrodes properly located and in firm skin contact?
- Is patient cable damaged?

Wandering or Irregular Baseline

- Is there excessive cable movement? This can be reduced by clipping to patient's clothing.
- Is the power cord on or near the monitor cable?
- Is there excessive movement by the patient? Muscle tremors from anxiety or shivering?
- Is site selection correct?
- Were proper skin preparation and application followed?
- Are the electrodes still moist?

Low-Amplitude Complexes

- Is size control adjusted properly?
- Were the electrodes applied properly?
- Is there dried gel on the electrodes?
- Change electrode sites. Check 12-lead ECG for lead with highest amplitude and attempt to simulate that lead.
- If none of the above steps remedies the problem, the weak signal may be the patient's normal complex.

Sixty-Cycle Interference

- Is the monitor size control set too high?
- Are there nearby electrical devices in use, especially poorly grounded ones?
- Were the electrodes applied properly?
- Is there dried gel on the electrodes?
- Are lead wires or connections damaged?

Electrocardiogram (ECG) Changes Associated With Electrolyte Imbalances

Electrolyte Imbalance	Major ECG Changes	Associated Dysrhythmias
Hyperkalemia	Tall, narrow, peaked T waves; flat, wide P waves; widening QRS	Sinus bradycardia; sinoatrial block; junctional rhythm; idioventricular rhythm; ventricular tachycardia; ventricular fibrillation
Hypokalemia	Prominent U waves; ST segment depression; T wave inversion	Ventricular premature beats; supraventricular tachycardia; ventricular tachycardia; ventricular fibrillation
Hypercalcemia	Shortened QT interval	Rare
Hypocalcemia	Lengthened QT interval; T wave lowering and inversion	Rare

Comparison of Second-Degree Atrioventricular (AV) Block

Mobitz I (Wenckebach)	Mobitz II
AV lesion is above bundle of His	Lesion is below bundle of His, in bundle branch system
Associated with inferior MI, digitalis toxicity, chronic lesion of conduction system	Associated with anterior MI, chronic lesion of conduction system
Described as ischemic, reversible, and transient in nature	Described as necrotic in nature
Dropped QRS complex preceded by progressive prolongation of the PR interval	Dropped QRS complex preceded by a fixed PR interval
Regular PP intervals	Regular PP intervals
QRS usually narrow	QRS usually wide
Usually responds well to pharmacologic intervention	Usually not responsive to pharmacologic intervention
May require temporary pacing in symptomatic patients	Often requires cardiac pacing

MI, myocardial infarction.
Adapted from Vinsant MO, Spence MI: Commonsense Approach to Coronary Care, 4th ed, p 310. St. Louis, CV Mosby, 1985.

Differential Diagnosis of Narrow QRS Tachycardia

Type of SVT	Onset	Atrial Rate	Ventricular Rate	RR Interval	Response to Carotid Massage
Sinus tachycardia	Gradual	100–180 beats/min	Same as sinus rate	Regular	Gradual slowing
PSVT	Abrupt	150–250 beats/min	Usually same as atrial; block seen with digitalis toxicity and AV node disease	Regular, except at onset and termination	May convert to NSR
Atrial flutter	Abrupt	250–350 beats/min	Occurs with 2:1, 3:1, 4:1, or varied ventricular response	Regular or regularly irregular	Abrupt slowing of ventricular response, flutter waves remain
Atrial fibrillation	Abrupt	400–650 beats/min	Depends on ability of AVN to conduct atrial impulse; decreased with drug therapy	Irregularly irregular	Abrupt slowing of ventricular response, fibrillation waves remain

SVT, supraventricular tachycardia; PSVT, paroxysmal supraventricular tachycardia; AV, atrioventricular; NSR, normal sinus rhythm; AVN, atrioventricular node.

*Approximate Normal Limits for QT Intervals in Seconds**

Heart Rate per Minute	Men and Children	Women
40	0.45–0.49	0.46–0.50
46	0.43–0.47	0.44–0.48
50	0.41–0.45	0.43–0.46
55	0.40–0.44	0.41–0.45
60	0.39–0.42	0.40–0.43
67	0.37–0.40	0.38–0.41
71	0.36–0.40	0.37–0.41
75	0.35–0.38	0.36–0.39
80	0.34–0.37	0.35–0.38
86	0.33–0.36	0.34–0.37
93	0.32–0.35	0.33–0.36
100	0.31–0.34	0.32–0.35
109	0.30–0.33	0.31–0.33
120	0.28–0.31	0.29–0.32
133	0.27–0.29	0.28–0.30
150	0.25–0.28	0.26–0.28
172	0.23–0.26	0.24–0.26

*Adapted from Frye SJ, Lounsbury P: Cardiac Rhythm Disorders: An Introduction Using the Nursing Process, p 38. Baltimore, Williams & Wilkins, 1988.

Identification of Bundle Branch Block on MCL$_1$ Tracing

RBBB
  1. QRS ≥ 0.12 sec
  2. rSR^1 configuration in V$_1$
LBBB
  1. QRS ≥ 0.12 sec
  2. Large negative qS or rS configuration in V$_1$

Commonly Used Antiarrhythmic Agents

Class	Action	Drug
I	All class I antiarrhythmic agents block sodium movement into the tissue, resulting in a reduced maximal velocity of phase 0 depolarization	
IA	Slows depolarization at all heart rates and increases the duration of action potential	Quinidine Procainamide Disopyramide
IB	Slows phase 0 depolarization at fast heart rates	Lidocaine Tocainamide Phenytoin Mexilitene
IC	Slows phase 0 depolarization at normal rates, does not affect the action potential duration	Encainide Flecainide Propafenone Moricizine
II	Blocks sympathetic stimulation of the conduction system	β-Blockers (propranolol) Acebutolol Esmolol
III	Prolongs the action potential duration	Amiodarone Bretylium Sotalol
IV	Blocks influx of calcium into the cell and decreases conduction velocity	Calcium channel blockers (verapamil, diltiazem)

Pharmacokinetics of Most Commonly Used Antiarrhythmic Drugs

Drug	Effect on ECG	Dose and Interval	Route	Adverse Effects	Therapeutic Plasma Level
Digoxin	Prolongs PR (±) ST depression	0.5 mg initially; 0.25 mg q2–4h total 1.0–1.5 mg first 24 hr	IV or PO	Nausea, vomiting, abdominal pain, blurred or colored vision, weakness, psychosis, VPCs, heart block	0.8–1.8 ng/ml
Quinidine	Prolongs QRS, QT, and PR (±)	100–600 mg q4–6h	PO	GI symptoms, cinchonism, thrombocytopenia, hypotension, heart block, ventricular tachycardia	2.3–5.0 μg/ml
Procainamide (Pronestyl)	Prolongs QRS, QT, and PR (±)	500 mg–1 g; then 2–5 g/day 250–500 mg q3–6 h 100 mg q5 m to 1 g total Maintenance: 2–4 mg/min	PO IM IV	GI symptoms, psychosis, hypotension, rash, lupus-like syndrome	4–10 μg/ml
Disopyramide (Norpace)	Prolongs QRS, QT, and PR	Loading: 200–300 mg Maintenance: 100–200 mg q6h	PO	Anticholinergic effects, hypotension, heart failure, heart block, tachyarrhythmias	2–8 μg/ml
Lidocaine	None	1 mg/kg; may repeat at 0.5 mg/kg	IV	Drowsiness, seizures	1.5–6 μg/ml
Propranolol (Inderal)	Prolongs PR, no change QRS, shortens QT	10–80 mg q6h 0.3–5 mg total (not >1 mg/min)	PO IV	Hypotension, heart failure, heart block, asthma	Not established; 50–100 ng/ml needed for β-blockade
Verapamil	Prolongs PR	5–10 mg 80–120 mg tid–qid	IV PO	Hypotension, bradycardia, dizziness, GI disturbance	Not established

ECG, electrocardiogram; VPC, ventricular premature contraction; GI, gastrointestinal.

Pharmacokinetics of Newer Antiarrhythmic Drugs

Drug	Effect on ECG	Dose and Interval	Route	Adverse Effects
Tocainide	No effect on PR, QRS, QT	400–600 mg q8h	Oral	Nausea, vomiting, abdominal pain, dizziness, tremor
Mexilitene	No effect on PR, QRS, QT	150–400 mg 3–4 times/day	Oral	Nausea, vomiting, dizziness, tremor
Encainide	Prolongs PR, QRS, may slightly prolong QT	25–50 mg q8h	Oral	Exacerbation of ventricular ectopy, visual disturbances, tremors, nausea
Flecainide	Prolongs PR, QRS, may slightly prolong QT	100–200 mg twice daily	Oral	Dizziness, blurred vision
Amiodarone	Prolongs QRS, QT; may slightly prolong PR	Loading dose—800–1200 mg/day for 10–14 days; then 200–400 mg/day	Oral	Corneal microdeposits, hyper/hypothyroidism, pulmonary fibrosis, skin sensitivity (blue skin), nausea, tremor, headache, ataxia
Bretylium	None	5–10 mg/kg	IV	Hypotension, nausea, vomiting
Propafenone	Prolongs PR and QRS	150–300 mg every 8 hr	Oral	Nausea, bitter taste, hypotension, exacerbation of ventricular ectopy
Moricizine	Prolongs PR and QRS	200–300 mg every 8 hr	Oral	Dizziness, headache, nausea, exacerbation of ventricular ectopy
Adenosine	Prolongs PR	6–12 mg	IV	Hypotension, facial flushing, dyspnea

ECG, electrocardiogram.

β-*Blocking Agents*

Drug	Cardioselective	Nonselective
Propranolol		X
Acebutolol	X	
Esmolol	X	
Atenolol	X	
Labetalol		X
Metoprolol	X	
Nadolol		X
Timolol		X

Comparison of Calcium Channel Blockers

	Nifedipine	Diltiazem	Verapamil	Amiodipine
Coronary blood flow	↑	↑	↑	↑
Myocardial O₂ demand	↓	↓	↓	↓
Vasodilate periphery	↓ ↓	↓	↓	↓ ↓
Cardiac output	↑	↑ ↓	↑ ↓	↑
Slow AV/SA conduction	No	Yes	Yes	No
Myocardial contractility	↓	↓	↓ ↓	↓

AV, atrioventricular; SA, sinoatrial.

Adapted from Frishman WH, Sonneblick EH: Calcium channel blockers. In Hurst JW, et al (eds): Heart, Arteries and Veins, p 1733. New York, McGraw-Hill, 1990.

Energy Requirements for Cardioversion

Indications	Energy in Joules (J)
Unstable VT with a pulse	50–360
Supraventricular tachycardia	75–100
Atrial flutter	25 initially
Atrial fibrillation	100 initially

VT, ventricular tachycardia.

Digitalis Preparations

Agent	Onset of Action (min)	Peak Effect (hr)	Average Half-life	Principal Excretory Path
Ouabain	5–10	$^{1}/_{2}$–2	21 hr	Renal; some GI
Digoxin	15–30	1–2	33 hr	Renal
Digitoxin	25–120	4–12	4–6 days	Hepatic

Agent	Average Digitalizing Dose		Usual Daily Oral Maintenance Dose
	Oral	IV	
Ouabain	—	0.3–0.5 mg	—
Digoxin	1.25–1.5	0.75–1.0 mg	0.25–0.5 mg
Digitoxin	0.7–1.2 mg	1.0 mg	0.1 mg

GI, gastrointestinal.

Manifestations of Digitalis Toxicity

Gastrointestinal

Anorexia
Vomiting
Abdominal pain
Diarrhea
Unexplained weight loss

Neurologic

Weakness
Blurred or colored vision
Psychosis

Cardiac (entirely manifest as dysrhythmias)

Atrial tachycardia, commonly with AV block
Junctional tachycardia
Ventricular ectopic rhythm
SA node depression
AV block
Bidirectional tachycardia

ACLS Guidelines
Universal Algorithm for Adult Emergency Cardiac Care

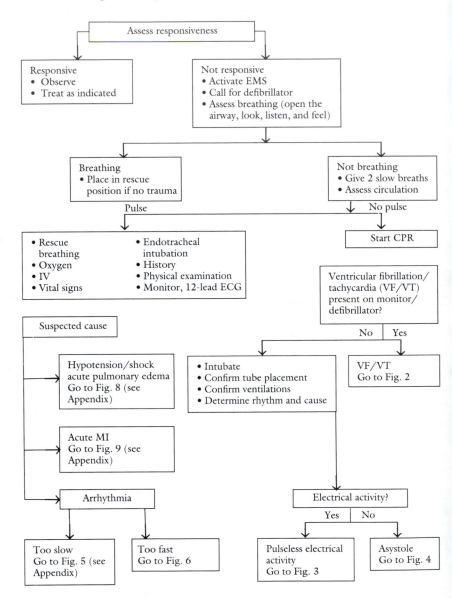

Fig. 1. Universal algorithm for adult emergency cardiac care (ECC). (JAMA 286[16]:2216.)

Algorithm for Ventricular Fibrillation and Pulseless Ventricular Tachycardia

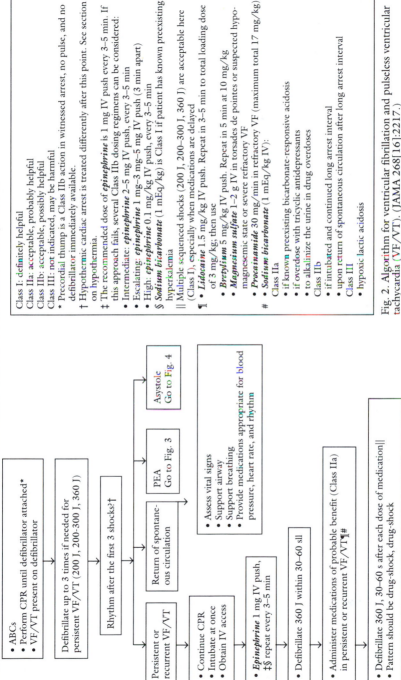

Class I: definitely helpful
Class IIa: acceptable, probably helpful
Class IIb: acceptable, possibly helpful
Class III: not indicated, may be harmful

* Precordial thump is a Class IIb action in witnessed arrest, no pulse, and no defibrillator immediately available.
† Hypothermic cardiac arrest is treated differently after this point. See section on hypothermia.
‡ The recommended dose of *epinephrine* is 1 mg IV push every 3–5 min. If this approach fails, several Class IIb dosing regimens can be considered:
• Intermediate: *epinephrine* 2–5 mg IV push, every 3–5 min
• Escalating: *epinephrine* 1 mg–3 mg–5 mg IV push (3 min apart)
• High: *epinephrine* 0.1 mg/kg IV push, every 3–5 min
§ *Sodium bicarbonate* (1 mEq/kg) is Class I if patient has known preexisting hyperkalemia
|| Multiple sequenced shocks (200 J, 200–300 J, 360 J) are acceptable here (Class I), especially when medications are delayed
¶ • *Lidocaine* 1.5 mg/kg IV push. Repeat in 3–5 min to total loading dose of 3 mg/kg; then use
  • *Bretylium* 5 mg/kg IV push. Repeat in 5 min at 10 mg/kg
  • *Magnesium sulfate* 1–2 g IV in torsades de pointes or suspected hypomagnesemic state or severe refractory VF
  • *Procainamide* 30 mg/min in refractory VF (maximum total 17 mg/kg):
  • *Sodium bicarbonate* (1 mEq/kg IV):
Class IIa
  • if known preexisting bicarbonate-responsive acidosis
  • if overdose with tricyclic antidepressants
  • to alkalinize the urine in drug overdoses
  Class IIb
  • if intubated and continued long arrest interval
  • upon return of spontaneous circulation after long arrest interval
  Class III
  • hypoxic lactic acidosis

Flowchart:

• ABCs
• Perform CPR until defibrillator attached*
• VF/VT present on defibrillator

Defibrillate up to 3 times if needed for persistent VF/VT (200 J, 200-300 J, 360 J)

Rhythm after the first 3 shocks?†

| Return of spontaneous circulation | PEA Go to Fig. 3 | Asystole Go to Fig. 4 |

• Assess vital signs
• Support airway
• Support breathing
• Provide medications appropriate for blood pressure, heart rate, and rhythm

Persistent or recurrent VF/VT

• Continue CPR
• Intubate at once
• Obtain IV access

• *Epinephrine* 1 mg IV push, ‡§ repeat every 3–5 min

• Defibrillate 360 J within 30–60 s||

• Administer medications of probable benefit (Class IIa) in persistent or recurrent VF/VT¶#

• Defibrillate 360 J, 30–60 s after each dose of medication||
• Pattern should be drug-shock, drug-shock

Fig. 2. Algorithm for ventricular fibrillation and pulseless ventricular tachycardia (VF/VT). (JAMA 268[16]:2217.)

Algorithm for Pulseless Electrical Activity

PEA includes
- Electromechanical dissociation (EMD)
- Pseudo-EMD
- Idioventricular rhythms
- Ventricular escape rhythms
- Bradyasystolic rhythms
- Postdefibrillation idioventricular rhythms

- Continue CPR
- Intubate at once
- Obtain IV access
- Assess blood flow using Doppler ultrasound

$\downarrow$

Consider possible causes
(Parentheses=possible therapies and treatments)
- Hypovolemia (volume infusion)
- Hypoxia (ventilation)
- Cardiac tamponade (pericardiocentesis)
- Tension pneumothorax (needle decompression)
- Hypothermia (see hypothermia algorithm, Section IV)
- Massive pulmonary embolism (surgery, *thrombolytics*)
- Drug overdoses such as tricyclics, digitalis, ß-blockers, calcium channel blockers
- Hyperkalemia*
- Acidosis†
- Massive acute myocardial infarction (go to Fig. 9; see Appendix)

$\downarrow$

- *Epinephrine* 1 mg IV push, *‡repeat every 3–5 min

$\downarrow$

- If absolute bradycardia (<60 beats/min) or relative bradycardia, give *atropine* 1 mg IV
- Repeat every 3–5 min up to a total of 0.04 mg/kg§

Class I: definitely helpful
Class IIa: acceptable, probably helpful
Class IIb: acceptable, possibly helpful
Class III: not indicated, may be harmful
Sodium bicarbonate 1 mEq/kg is Class I if patient has known preexisting hyperkalemia.
† *Sodium bicarbonate* 1 mEq/kg:
  Class IIa
  - if known preexisting bicarbonate-responsive acidosis
  - if overdose with tricyclic antidepressants
  - to alkalinize the urine in drug overdoses
  Class IIb
  - if intubated and long arrest interval
  - upon return of spontaneous circulation after long arrest interval
  Class III
  - hypoxic lactic acidosis
‡The recommended dose of *epinephrine* is 1 mg IV push every 3–5 min.
  If this approach fails, several Class IIb dosing regimens can be considered.
  - Intermediate: *epinephrine* 2–5 mg IV push, every 3–5 min
  - Escalating: *epinephrine* 1 mg–3 mg–5 mg IV push (3 min apart)
  - High: *epinephrine* 0.1 mg/kg IV push, every 3–5 min
  §Shorter *atropine* dosing intervals are possibly helpful in cardiac arrest (Class IIb).

Fig. 3. Algorithm for pulseless electrical activity (PEA) (electromechanical dissociation [EMD]). (JAMA 268[16]:2219.)

Asystole Treatment Algorithm

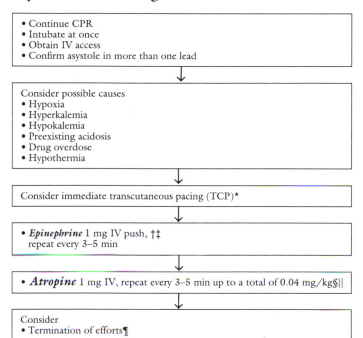

- Continue CPR
- Intubate at once
- Obtain IV access
- Confirm asystole in more than one lead

↓

Consider possible causes
- Hypoxia
- Hyperkalemia
- Hypokalemia
- Preexisting acidosis
- Drug overdose
- Hypothermia

↓

Consider immediate transcutaneous pacing (TCP)*

↓

- *Epinephrine* 1 mg IV push, †‡
  repeat every 3–5 min

↓

- *Atropine* 1 mg IV, repeat every 3–5 min up to a total of 0.04 mg/kg§‖

↓

Consider
- Termination of efforts¶

Class I: definitely helpful
Class IIa: acceptable, probably helpful
Class IIb: acceptable, possibly helpful
Class III: not indicated, may be harmful
* TCP is a Class IIb intervention. Lack of success may be due to delays in pacing. To be
  effective TCP must be performed early, simultaneously with drugs. Evidence does not
  support routine use of TCP for asystole.
†The recommended dose of *epinephrine* is 1 mg IV push every 3–5 min. If this approach fails,
  several Class IIb dosing regimens can be considered:
  - Intermediate: *epinephrine* 2–5 mg IV push, every 3–5 min
  - Escalating: *epinephrine* 1 mg–3 mg–5 mg IV push (3 min apart)
  - High: *epinephrine* 0.1 mg/kg IV push, every 3–5 min
‡ *Sodium bicarbonate* 1 mEq/kg is Class I if patient has known preexisting hyperkalemia.
§ Shorter *atropine* dosing intervals are Class IIb in asystolic arrest.
‖ *Sodium bicarbonate* 1 mEq/kg:
  Class IIa
  - if known preexisting bicarbonate-responsive acidosis
  - if overdose with tricyclic antidepressants
  - to alkalinize the urine in drug overdoses
  Class IIb
  - if intubated and continued long arrest interval
  - upon return of spontaneous circulation after long arrest interval
  Class III
  - hypoxic lactic acidosis
¶ If patient remains in asystole or other agonal rhythms after successful intubation and initial
  medications and no reversible causes are identified, consider termination of resuscitative
  efforts by a physician. Consider interval since arrest.

Fig. 4. Asystole treatment algorithm. (JAMA 286[16]:2220.)

Tachycardia Algorithm

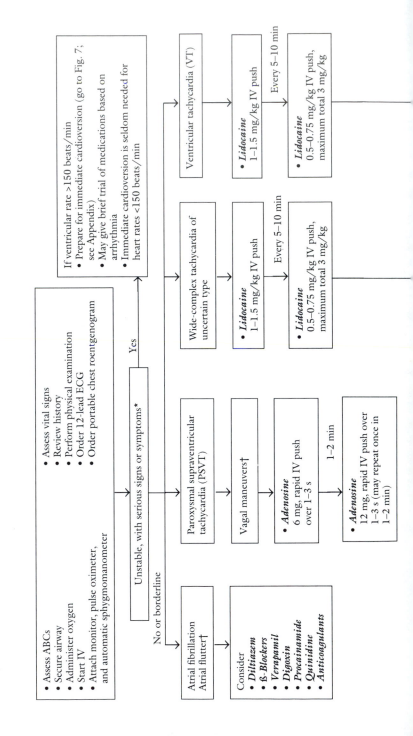

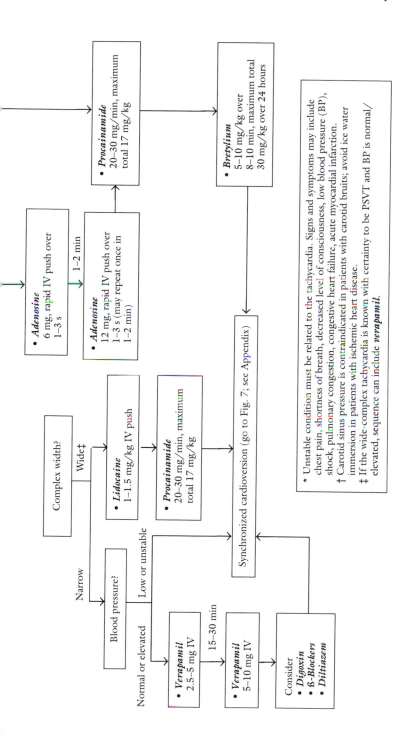

Fig. 6. Tachycardia algorithm. (JAMA 268[16]:2223.)

The flowchart contains the following elements:

Complex width?

Narrow — Wide‡

Wide‡:
- *Lidocaine* 1–1.5 mg/kg IV push
- *Procainamide* 20–30 mg/min, maximum total 17 mg/kg
- Synchronized cardioversion (go to Fig. 7; see Appendix)

Narrow — Blood pressure?

Normal or elevated — Low or unstable

Normal or elevated:
- *Verapamil* 2.5–5 mg IV
- 15–30 min
- *Verapamil* 5–10 mg IV
- Consider
  - *Digoxin*
  - *ß-Blockers*
  - *Diltiazem*

- *Adenosine* 6 mg, rapid IV push over 1–3 s
- 1–2 min
- *Adenosine* 12 mg, rapid IV push over 1–3 s (may repeat once in 1–2 min)
- *Procainamide* 20–30 mg/min, maximum total 17 mg/kg
- *Bretylium* 5–10 mg/kg over 8–10 min, maximum total 30 mg/kg over 24 hours

* Unstable condition must be related to the tachycardia. Signs and symptoms may include chest pain, shortness of breath, decreased level of consciousness, low blood pressure (BP), shock, pulmonary congestion, congestive heart failure, acute myocardial infarction.

† Carotid sinus pressure is contraindicated in patients with carotid bruits; avoid ice water immersion in patients with ischemic heart disease.

‡ If the wide-complex tachycardia is known with certainty to be PSVT and BP is normal/ elevated, sequence can include *verapamil.*

ICHD Code for Differentiation of Pacemaker Functional Capabilities

Paced Chamber	Sensing Chamber	Response to Sensing
V = Ventricle	V = Ventricle	I = Inhibited
A = Atrium	A = Atrium	T = Triggered
D = Dual chambers	D = Dual	D = Dual
O = None	O = None	O = None

Programmable Function	Special Antitachycardia Functions
P = Program (rate and/or output)	P = Standard pacer technology
M = Multiprogrammable	S = Shock
C = Communicating.	D = Paces and shocks
R = Rate modulation	
O = None	

Commonly Used Pacemaker Modes

Although the VVI (ventricular demand) pacemaker is the mode most commonly used in temporary pacing, other modes will be encountered by the critical care nurse due to advances in dual chambered temporary pacing and the multiprogrammability in permanent pacemakers.

Teaching the Patient With a Pacemaker

1. Knowledge of Condition

- Elicit the patient's previous knowledge of pacemakers and clarify any misconceptions.
- If appropriate, clarify the difference between heart block and heart attack. (A patient may confuse cardiac monitoring with pacing and become very anxious when the monitoring electrodes are removed.)
- Don't assume *anything* about the patient's understanding.
- The anatomy of the heart should be discussed in general terms when explaining the need for pacing and how the pacemaker takes the place of or complements spontaneous rhythm.
- The difference between temporary and permanent pacing also should be discussed.

2. Patient Activity

- Passive and active range-of-motion exercises should be started on the affected arm 48 hr after pacemaker implantation in the pectoralis major muscle to avoid "frozen shoulder."
- The patient should be instructed to repeat these exercises several times daily until the implantation site is completely free of discomfort through all ranges of arm motion.
- Explain that the pacemaker is relatively sturdy and that touching or bathing the implantation site will not damage it.
- The patient's activities of daily living and recreational activities should be discussed *before* permanent pacing to ascertain an appropriate site for implantation; for example, the right pectoralis muscle should not be used in the right-handed rifle hunter.
- Abdominal implantation may be preferable for the avid swimmer because of the strenuous arm activity.
- Activities that may result in high impact or stress at the implantation site should be avoided. This includes all contact sports.
- Instruct the patient to report any activity that may have damaged his pacemaker.
- The patient can return to work at the discretion of his physician.
- Discuss the type of work he will do and what his job entails. He may return to whatever degree of sexual activity he prefers.
- The patient should be aware that his pacemaker may set off the alarm on metal-detector devices in airports.

3. Signs of Pacemaker Malfunction

- The symptoms of pacemaker malfunction are those associated with decreased perfusion of the brain, heart, or skeletal muscles.
- The patient should be instructed to report any dizziness, fainting, chest pain, shortness of breath, undue fatigue, or fluid retention.
- Fluid retention should be described in terms of sudden weight gain, "puffy ankles," "tightness of rings," and so forth.

(continued)

Teaching the Patient With a Pacemaker (continued)

---

3. Signs of Pacemaker Malfunction (*continued*)

- Patient should be instructed to take pulse once daily upon awakening. Patient should report a pulse rate that is more than 5 beats/min slower than that at which pacemaker is set.
- Patient should be aware that pulse may be somewhat irregular if it is a demand pacemaker and has some spontaneous beats as well as paced beats. It must be stressed that this does not signify pacemaker malfunction.

4. Signs of Infection

- The patient should report any redness, swelling, drainage, or increase in soreness at the implantation site.

5. Pulse Generator Replacement

- Instruct the patient regarding the expected life of pacemaker battery.
- Patient should know that generator replacement requires hospitalization for about 1 day and that usually only the generator will need to be replaced.

6. Medications

- The patient should be instructed regarding any medication needed.
- Patient should know the name of the medication, as well as the dose, frequency of administration, side effects, and use of each medication.

7. Safety Measures

- The patient should inform any physician or dentist of the pacemaker and of the medications being taken.
- Patient should carry a pacemaker identification card at all times. This card shows the brand and model of pacemaker, the date of insertion, and the programmed settings.
- It also is advisable to wear a medical alert bracelet or necklace stating that patient has a pacemaker.

8. Follow-up Care

- The importance of physician or clinic follow-up visits should be stressed.
- The follow-up visit will include an interval history and physical examination and a 12-lead ECG.
- Many pacemaker clinics have specialized equipment available to measure the rate, amplitude, duration, and contours of the pacemaker artifact. This information is very helpful in predicting battery depletion. Some clinics have the capability for obtaining this information by telephone, reducing the necessity for travel to the clinic.

Direct Physiological Effects of IABP

Inflation

↑ aortic diastolic pressure
↑ aortic root pressure
↑ coronary perfusion pressure
↑ oxygen supply

Deflation

↓ aortic end-diastolic pressure
↓ impedance to ejection
↓ afterload
↓ oxygen demand

Indications for IABP

- Cardiogenic shock after acute infarction
- Left ventricular failure in the postoperative cardiac surgery patient
- Severe unstable angina
- Postinfarction ventricular septal defect or mitral regurgitation
- Septic shock
- General surgery for the patient with cardiovascular disease
- Bridge to cardiac transplantation

Contraindications to IABP

- Aortic valve incompetence
- Severe peripheral vascular occlusive disease
- Previous aortofemoral or aortoiliac bypass grafts
- Aortic aneurysm

Calculation of Inflation Time for a Heart Rate of 60

msec in RR interval

$$+ \; \frac{60,000 \text{ msec/min}}{\text{patient's heart rate (60 beats/min)}}$$

one RR interval = 1,000 msec
systole ($^{1}/_{3}$) ~ 400 msec
diastole ($^{2}/_{3}$) ~ 600 msec

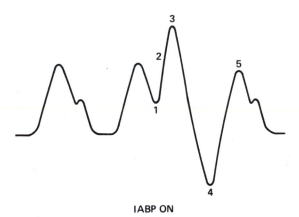

IABP ON

Inspection of the arterial waveform with intra-aortic balloon assistance should include observation of (1) inflation point; (2) inflation slope; (3) diastolic peak pressure; (4) end-diastolic dip; (5) next systolic peak.

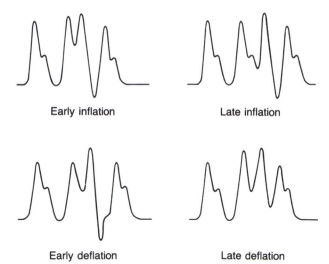

Early inflation   Late inflation

Early deflation   Late deflation

Illustration of possible errors occurring with timing.

Criteria for Assessment of Effective IABP on the Arterial Pressure Waveform

- Inflation occurs at the dicrotic notch.
- Inflation slope is parallel to the systolic upstroke and is a straight line.
- Diastolic augmentation peak is greater than or equal to the preceding systolic peak.
- An end-diastolic dip in pressure is created with balloon deflation.
- The following systolic peak (assisted systole) is lower than the preceding systole (unassisted systole).

Indications for Weaning From IABP

- Hemodynamic stability
  Cardiac index >2 L/min
  PCWP <20 mm Hg
  Systolic blood pressure >100 mm Hg
- Minimal requirements for vasopressor support
- Evidence of adequate cardiac function
  Good peripheral pulses
  Adequate urine output
  Absence of pulmonary edema
  Improved mentation
- Evidence of good coronary perfusion
  Absence of ventricular ectopy
  Absence of ischemia on the ECG
- Severe vascular insufficiency
- Balloon leakage
- Deteriorating, irreversible condition

Approaches to Weaning From IABP

- Gradually decrease assist ratio
- Decrease diastolic augmentation

Troubleshooting Arterial Pressure Monitoring

Problem	Cause	Prevention	Treatment
Damped pressure tracing	Catheter tip against vessel wall	Usually cannot be avoided	Pull catheter hub back
			Rotate or reposition extremity while observing pressure waveform
	Partial occlusion of catheter tip by clot	Use continuous flush device	Aspirate clot with syringe and manually flush system with heparinized flush solution
		Maintain heparinized saline flush solution under pressure (>300 mm Hg)	
	Clotting in stopcock or transducer	Thoroughly flush catheter after blood withdrawal	Flush stopcock and transducer; if no improvement, change stopcock and transducer
		Use continuous flush device	
Abnormally high or low readings	Change in transducer level	Maintain transducer at midchest level for serial pressure measurements	Recheck patient and transducer positions

(continued)

Troubleshooting Arterial Pressure Monitoring *(continued)*

Problem	Cause	Prevention	Treatment
Damped pressure without improvement after flushing	Air bubbles in transducer or connecting tubing	Carefully flush transducer and tubing when setting up system and attaching to catheter	Check system; flush manually; flush air bubbles out of transducer
	Nonpressure tubing used	Use stiff, short pressure tubing	Shorten tubing or replace softer tubing with stiff pressure tubing
No pressure available	Transducer not open to catheter	Follow routine, systematic steps for setting up system and turning stopcocks	Check system—stopcocks, monitor/amplifier setup
	Monitor/amplifier off		
	Incorrect scale selection on monitor	Select scale appropriate to expected range of pressure to be measured	Select appropriate scale

From Daily EK, Schroeder JS: Techniques in Bedside Hemodynamic Monitoring, 4th ed. St. Louis, CV Mosby, 1989.

Autotransfusion Troubleshooting Guidelines

Complication	Cause	Intervention
Coagulation	Insufficient anticoagulant added	Added regional anticoagulant such as CPD at a ratio of 7:1 blood to CPD
		Shake collection device periodically to mix blood and regional anticoagulant
	Mediastinal blood not defibrinogenated	Check reversal of anticoagulant
		Strip chest tubes PRN
Hemolysis	Blood trauma secondary to turbulence or roller pumps	Avoid skimming operative field during blood harvesting
		Avoid using equipment containing roller pumps
		Maintain vacuum below 30 mm Hg when collecting blood from chest tubes, below 60 mm Hg when aspirating from a surgical site
Coagulopathies	Hypothermia, shock, multiple transfusions	Patients autotransfused with more than 4,000 ml of blood may require transfusion of fresh frozen plasma or platelet concentrate
	Decreased levels of platelets and fibrinogen	
	Platelets trapped in filters	
	Increased levels of fibrin split products	

(continued)

Autotransfusion Troubleshooting Guidelines (*continued*)

Complication	Cause	Intervention
Particulate and air emboli	Microaggregate debris	Use 20 to 40 μm microaggregate filter during reinfusion
	Air emboli	Use only infusion pumps with a bubble detector system
		Remove air from blood bags prior to reinfusion
	Nonparenteral medication at site	Avoid use of blood containing non-IV medications
		Wash blood as indicated
Sepsis	Breakdown of aseptic technique	Broad-spectrum antibiotics as indicated
		Maintain good aseptic technique
		Reinfuse within 4 to 6 hr of initial collection
	Contaminated blood	Avoid use of blood from infected areas and/or with known contaminants, such as stool and urine
Citrate toxicity (rare and unpredicable)	Chelating effect of citrate in the CPD/ACD on calcium	Monitor for hypotension, dysrhythmias, and myocardial contractility; when more than 2,000 ml of CPD anticoagulated blood is given over a 20-min period, calcium chloride may be given prophylactically
	Hyperkalemia, hypocalcemia, acidosis, hypothermia, myocardial dysfunction, and liver or renal dysfunction are disposing factors	Slow down or stop CPD infusion, correct acidosis
		Monitor toxicity with frequent blood gases and serum calcium levels

CPD, citrate–phosphate–dextrose; ACD, acid–citrate–dextrose.

Contraindications to Autotransfusion

- Malignant neoplasm
- Infections and infestations
- Blood contamination
- Coagulopathies
- Excessive hemolysis
- Renal failure

Diagnostic Tests Used to Detect Myocardial Ischemia

Procedure	Abnormal Findings	Special Considerations
Standard 12-Lead ECG*	Transient ST segment and T wave changes in patients with chest pain at rest or of prolonged duration	
Holter monitoring	Transient ST segment and T wave changes occurring at rest or with activity	Only two ECG leads monitored
Stress echocardiogram	Segmental wall motion abnormality associated with echocardiogram obtained during exercise	May be used in patients with ventricular conduction defects Pharmacologic agents may be used in patients who cannot exercise
Exercise ECG	Transient ST segment and T wave changes occurring with exercise	Cannot be used in patients who are unable to exercise or who have left bundle or paced rhythm Does not provide good information on the location of the coronary artery disease
Radionuclide perfusion stress study	"Cold spot" image or perfusion defect associated with scan obtained during exercise	May be used in patients with ventricular conduction defects Pharmacologic agents may be used in patients who cannot exercise

*ECG, electrocardiogram.

Specific Electrocardiogram (ECG) Changes for Acute Transmural Myocardial Infarctions

Infarct Area	ECG Changes
Anterior	ST segment elevation in leads V_3–V_4; reciprocal changes (ST depression) in leads II, III, aVF (Fig. 12–3)
Inferior	ST segment elevation in leads II, III, aVF; reciprocal changes (ST depression) in V_1–V_6, I, aVL (Fig. 12–5)
Lateral	ST segment elevation in I, aVL, V_5–V_6 (Fig. 12–4)
Posterior	Reciprocal changes in II, III, aVF; predominant R waves in V_1–V_2
Right ventricle	Mimic inferior wall changes

Hemodynamic Assessment of the Myocardial Infarction

Pulmonary Capillary Wedge Pressure (mm Hg)	Cardiac Index (L/min/m²)	Clinical State	Anticipated Therapy
<18	>2.2	Normal	Reduced metabolic needs
<18	<2.2	Volume depletion	Volume expansion with crystalloids
>18	>2.2	Pulmonary congestion	Diuretics Nitrates
>18	<2.2	Cardiogenic shock	Vasopressors Inotropic agents Afterload reducers IAPB

IAPB, intra-aortic balloon pump.

Cardiac Enzymes After Acute Myocardial Infarction

	Increase	Peak	Return to Normal
CK	3–8 hr	10–30 hr	2–3 days
CK-MB	3–6 hr	10–24 hr	2–3 days
CK-MB$_2$	1–6 hr	4–8 hr	12–48 hr
LDH	14–24 hr	48–72 hr	7–14 days
LDH$_1$	14–24 hr	48–72 hr	7–14 days

Patient Selection Criteria for Thrombolytic Therapy

Inclusion by Symptoms

- Recent onset (<6 hr) of acute MI symptoms
- Pain; chest pain that may radiate to arm, jaw, neck, or back
- ECG: evidence of an acute MI, ST segment elevation

Exclusion by History

- Recent major surgery (<10 days)
- Recent trauma (<10 days)
- CVA (within 2 months)
- Recent gastrointestinal or genitourinary bleeding (<10 days)
- Severe hypertension (≥180/110 mm Hg)
- Acute pericarditis
- Subacute bacterial endocarditis
- Recent streptococcal infection (<6 months)
- Pregnancy
- Severe liver dysfunction
- Hemorrhagic ophthalmic disease
- Aortic dissection
- Age over 75 years
- Oral anticoagulant therapy
- Previous SK or APSAC therapy (<1 year)

MI, myocardial infarction; ECG, electrocardiogram; CVA, cerebrovascular accident; SK, streptokinase; APSAC, anisoylated plasminogen streptokinase activator.

From TIMI II: Comparison of invasive and conservative strategies after treatment with IV t-PA in acute MI. N Engl J Med 320:618–627, 1989.

Comparison of Approved Thrombolytic Agents

	SK	t-PA	APSAC
Dose	1.5 million units in 60 minutes	6–10 mg bolus initially, 50 mg: first hour 20 mg: second hour 20 mg: third hour (Dose may be varied if weight is ≤65 kg)	30 units in 2–5 min
Half-life	23 min	5 min	90 min
Blood clearance	Hours	30–40 min	4–6 hr
Cost (per treatment)	$390	$2,200	$1,700
Variance in complications		Highest reocclusion rates	Highest allergic rate; highest hypotensive rates

SK, streptokinase; t-PA, tissue plasminogen activator; APSAC, anisoylated plasminogen streptokinase activator.

Adapted from Daily EK: Clinical management of patients receiving thrombolytic therapy. Heart Lung 20: 559–565, 1991.

Signs and Symptoms of Left Ventricular Failure

- Pulmonary vascular congestion
- Dyspnea
- Orthopnea
- Paroxysmal nocturnal dyspnea (PND)
- Irritating cough
- Acute pulmonary edema
- Decreased cardiac output
- Atrial gallop—S_4
- Ventricular gallop—S_3
- Lung crackles
- Dysrhythmias
- Wheezing breath sounds
- Pulsus alternans
- Weight gain
- Cheyne–Stokes respirations
- Radiographic evidence of pulmonary vascular congestion

Signs and Symptoms of Right Ventricular Failure

- Low cardiac output
- Jugular vein distention
- Dependent edema
- Dysrhythmias
- Right ventricular S_3 and S_4
- Hyperresonance with percussion
- Low immobile diaphragms
- Decreased breath sounds
- Increased anteroposterior chest diameter

Sample Continuum of Patient/Family Educational Goals After Acute MI

When mastery of content is to be expected:	Acute Phase	Before ICU Discharge	At Hospital Discharge
Pathophysiology of heart disease	Can identify angina, using 1–10 scale for reference	Can initiate treatment of angina (rest, NTG, O$_2$ use)	Knowledgeable about medications, when to seek medical assistance
Environment of hospital	Understands procedures	Asks appropriate questions	Knowledgeable about disease process and therapy
Lifestyle modifications	Complies with activity limitations Complies with dietary limitations	Can state relationship between activity and cardiac work load Begins light activity States risk factors Selects appropriate meals	Can progress activity as tolerated Placement in cardiac rehabilitation program Can state dietary restrictions
Treatment of disease	Accepts medications as ordered	Can identify medications Can identify risk factors	Knowledgeable about medications, dose, timing, action, and side effects Plans for risk factor reduction Begins cardiac rehabilitation program
Emotional adaptation	Accepts sedation to minimize stress	Begins to communicate about lifestyle changes Becomes involved with resolving emotions related to surviving a critical illness	Involves self and loved ones in plans for lifestyle changes Expresses feelings Participates in group recovery program

Indications and Contraindications for PTCA

Indications	Contraindications
Clinical	
Symptomatic (angina unrelieved by medical therapy)	Presence of coronary artery spasm
Asymptomatic but with severe underlying stenosis	
Stable/unstable angina	
Acute myocardial infarction	
High-risk surgical candidates	
Anatomic	
Severe stenosis (≥50%)	Mild stenosis (<50%)
Proximal and distal lesions	Diffuse "cheesy" atheroma in grafts
Single and multivessel disease	Evidence of preexisting dissection or thrombosis
Bifurcation lesions	"Unprotected" left main coronary artery
Ostial lesions	
Totally occluded vessels	
Bypass graft lesions	
"Protected" left main coronary artery (previous LAD or CIRC CABG)	

LAD, left anterior descending artery; CIRC, circumflex artery; CABG, coronary artery bypass graft.

Summary of Medications Most Often Associated With PTCA and PBV

Anticoagulants/Antiplatelets

Aspirin

Indications: Prophylaxis of coronary and cerebral arterial thrombus formation
Actions: Blocks platelet aggregation
Dosage: 80–325 mg qid
Adverse effects: Well tolerated. Nausea, vomiting, diarrhea, headache, and vertigo occasionally

Dipyridamole (Persantine)

Indications:
1. Unstable angina pectoris
2. Prophylaxis in thromboembolic disease by decreasing platelet aggregation
Actions: Antiplatelet effect, mild vasodilatation
Dosage: 25–75 mg tid
Adverse effects: Well tolerated. Nausea, vomiting, diarrhea, headache, and vertigo occasionally

Heparin

Indications: Prophylaxis of impending coronary occlusion and prophylaxis of peripheral arterial embolism
Actions: Inhibits clotting of blood and formation of fibrin clots. Inactivates thrombin, preventing conversion of fibrinogen to fibrin. Also prevents formation of a stable fibrin clot by inhibiting the activation of fibrin stabilizing factor. Inhibits reactions that lead to clotting but does not alter normal components of blood. Prolongs clotting time but does not affect bleeding time. Does not lyse clots.
Dosage: Varies with indications. IV or IA: 10,000 U at start of PTCA
Adverse effects: Uncontrollable bleeding, hypersensitivity

Sulfinpyrazone (Anturane)

Indications: Prophylaxis in thromboembolic disease
Actions: Blocks platelet aggregation
Dosage: 100–200 mg qid
Adverse effects: GI irritation (lessened if taken in divided doses with meals), hypersensitivity (rash and fever), blood dyscrasias

Coronary Vasodilators

Isosorbide dinitrate (Isordil, Sorbitrate)

Indications: Prophylaxis of angina
Actions: A nitrate that acts as a smooth muscle relaxant. Causes coronary vasodilation without increasing myocardial oxygen consumption. Secondary to general vasodilation, blood pressure decreases.

(*continued*)

Summary of Medications Most Often Associated With
PTCA and PBV (continued)

Dosage:
1. Sublingual: 2.5–10 mg q2–3 h prn angina
2. Oral: 5–40 mg qid
3. Sustained action oral: 40 mg q6–12 h
Adverse effects:
1. Cutaneous vasodilation that can cause flushing
2. Headache, transient dizziness, and weakness
3. Excessive hypotension

Nitroglycerin

Indications: Control of blood pressure and angina pectoris
Actions: Potent vasodilator that affects primarily the venous system. Selectively dilates large coronary arteries increasing blood flow to ischemic subendocardium.
Dosage:
1. Sublingual: 0.3–0.4 mg prn chest pain
2. Topical (patch): 2.5–10 mg/day. Indicated for primary, secondary, or nocturnal angina due to more sustained effect.
3. IV: 5 μg/min to start—titrate to patient response. (No fixed dose due to variable response in different patients.)
Adverse effects:
1. Excessive and prolonged hypotension
2. Headache
3. Tachycardia, palpitations
4. Nausea, vomiting, apprehension
5. Retrosternal discomfort

Calcium Channel Blockers

Nifedipine, Diltiazem

Indications:
1. Angina pectoris due to coronary artery spasm and fixed vessel disease
2. Hypertension
3. Dysrhythmias
Actions: Inhibits calcium ion flux across the cell membrane of the cardiac muscle and vascular smooth muscle without changing serum calcium concentration. Decreases afterload through peripheral arterial dilation and
1. Reduces systemic and pulmonary vascular resistance
2. Vasodilates coronary circulation
3. Decreases myocardial oxygen demands and increases myocardial oxygen supply
Dosage:
1. Nefidipine (Procardia): 10–30 mg tid-qid
2. Diltiazem (Cardizem): 30–90 mg tid-qid

(*continued*)

Summary of Medications Most Often Associated With PTCA and PBV (continued)

Adverse effects:
1. Contraindicated in patients with sick sinus syndrome
2. Hypertension after IV use
3. GI distress
4. Headache, vertigo, flushing
5. Peripheral edema, occasional increase in angina, tachycardia

Vasopressors

Levophed (norepinephrine)

Indications: Restoration of a normal systemic blood pressure in acute hypotensive states
Actions: α-Adrenergic action causes an increase in systolic and diastolic pressures. Peripheral vascular resistance also increases in most vascular beds and blood flow is reduced through the liver, kidney, and usually skeletal muscle.
Dosage: IV concentration: 2 mg Levophed/250 ml solution. Initial IV infusion of 2–3 ml (8–12 μg/min), adjust rate of infusion to reestablish and maintain a normal blood pressure (80–100 mm Hg) sufficient to maintain blood flow to vital organs.
Note: Before administering, hypovolemia should be corrected.
Adverse effects:
1. Anxiety, bradycardia, severe hypertension, marked increase in peripheral vascular resistance, headache, decreased cardiac input
2. Necrosis and sloughing can occur with extravasation at infusion site.
3. Reduced blood flow to vital organs (kidney, liver)

See text for full discussion of antiarrhythmics.
PTCA, percutaneous transluminal coronary angioplasty; PBV, percutaneous balloon valvuloplasty; GI, gastrointestinal.

Complications of PTCA

Complications	General Signs/ Symptoms	Possible Interventions
Prolonged angina	Angina pectoris	CABG
Myocardial infarction	Dysrhythmias: tachycardia, bradycardia, ventricular tachycardia/ fibrillation	Redo PTCA Oxygen
Abrupt reclosure		Medications: vasodilators (nitrates), calcium channel blockers, analgesics, anticoagulants, vasopressors
Dissection/intimal tear	Marked hypotension	
	Acute ECG changes (ST segment change)	
Hypotension	Nausea/vomiting	
Coronary branch occlusion	Pallor	
Coronary thrombosis	Restlessness	Complete bed rest
	Cardiac/respiratory arrest	Increase IV fluid volume within patient tolerance
Restenosis	Angina pectoris	Redo PTCA
	Positive exercise test	CABG
Marked change in heart rate: bradycardia, ventricular tachycardia, ventricular fibrillation	Rate below 60/min	Temporary pacemaker
	Rate above 250/min	Defibrillation
	No discernible cardiac rhythm	Medications: antiarrhythmics, vasopressors
	Pallor	
	Loss of consciousness	
	Hypotension	
Vascular: excessive blood loss	Hypotension	Possible surgical repair
	Decreased urine output (from hypovolemia)	Fluids
	Decreased hemoglobin/ hematocrit	Transfusion
	Pallor	Oxygen
	Hematoma at puncture site	Flat in bed or in Trendelenburg position

(*continued*)

Complications of PTCA *(continued)*

Complications	General Signs/Symptoms	Possible Interventions
Allergic	Hypotension, urticaria, nausea/vomiting, hives, laryngospasm, erythema, shortness of breath	Medications: antihistamines, steroids, antiemetics Clear liquids/NPO Oxygen With anaphylaxis: fluids for volume expansion, epinephrine, vasopressors for hypotension
Central nervous system events	Changes in level of consciousness Hemiparesis Hypoventilation/respiratory depression	Oxygen Discontinue/hold sedatives Medication: narcotic antagonist as a respiratory stimulant

Miscellaneous complications: conduction defects, pulmonary embolism, pulmonary edema, coronary air embolism, respiratory arrest, febrile episode, nausea, minor bleeding.

PTCA, percutaneous transluminal coronary angioplasty; CABG, coronary artery bypass graft; ECG, electrocardiogram.

Preoperative Teaching of the Cardiac Surgery Patient: The Critical Care Unit Experience

1. Equipment, tubes, and lines used in critical care
   a. Cardiac monitor
   b. Arterial line
   c. Thermodilution catheter
   d. IVs and IV infusion pumps
   e. Endotracheal tube and ventilator
      1. Suctioning
      2. Inability to talk
      3. How to communicate when intubated
      4. When extubation can be anticipated
   f. Foley catheter
   g. Chest tubes
   h. Pacing wires
   i. Nasogastric tube
   j. Soft hand restraints
2. Incisions and dressings
   a. Median sternotomy incision
   b. Leg incision (is saphenous vein is used)
3. Patient's immediate postoperative appearance
   a. Skin yellow due to use of Betadine solution in operating room
   b. Skin pale and cool to touch due to hypothermia during surgery
   c. Generalized "puffiness" especially noticeable in neck, face, and hands due to third spacing of fluid given during cardiopulmonary bypass

4. Process of awakening from anesthesia
   a. Patient recovers in the critical care unit; does not go to the postanesthesia care unit
   b. Sensations patient will feel
   c. Noises patient will hear
   d. May be aware or able to hear but unable to respond
5. Discomfort from incision, chest tubes, and endotracheal tube
   a. Amount of discomfort to be expected
   b. When pain might be expected
   c. Relief mechanisms
      a. Positioning/splinting
      b. Medications
6. Postoperative respiratory care
   a. Turning
   b. Effective coughing and deep breathing after extubation
   c. Use of pillow to splint median sternotomy incision
   d. Incentive spirometry
   e. Have patient practice b, c, and d preoperatively
7. Postoperative activity progression
8. Visiting policy in critical care area

Effects of Cardiopulmonary Bypass

Causes	Clinical Implications
Increased Capillary Permeability	
Interface between blood and nonphysiological surfaces or bypass circuit leads to	Large amounts of fluid move from the intravascular to the interstitial space during and up to 6 h after cardiopulmonary bypass.
• Complement activation that increases capillary permeability;	Patient becomes edematous.
• Platelet activation—platelets secrete vasoactive substances that increase capillary permeability;	
• Release of other vasoactive substances that increase capillary permeability.	
Hemodilution	
Solution used to prime extracorporeal circuit dilutes patient's blood.	Decreased blood viscosity improves capillary perfusion during nonpulsatile flow and hypothermia.
Secretion of vasopressin (ADH) is increased.	Hgb and Hct decrease.
Levels of renin–angiotensin–aldosterone are increased because of nonpulsatile renal perfusion.	Levels of coagulation factors are decreased because of dilution.
Total body water is increased.	Intravascular colloid osmotic pressure is decreased, contributing to movement of fluid from intravascular to interstitial spaces.
	Water is retained at collecting tubule of kidney.
	Aldosterone causes retention of sodium and water at renal tubule.
	Weight gain occurs.

Alterations in Coagulation

Procoagulant effects:

- Interface between blood and nonendothelial surfaces of bypass circuit activates intrinsic coagulation cascade.
- Platelet damage activates intrinsic pathway.

Risk of microemboli is increased.

Anticoagulant effects:

- Interface between blood and nonendothelial surfaces of bypass circuit causes platelets to adhere to tubing and to clump; abnormal platelet function; activation of coagulation cascade, which depletes clotting factors; denaturization of plasma proteins, including coagulation factors.
- Coagulation factors decreased as a result of hemodilution.
- Heparin and protamine.

Platelet count decreases by 50% to 70% of baseline.
Abnormal postoperative bleeding occurs.
Possibility of bleeding diathesis exists.

Damage to Blood Cells

Exposure of blood to nonendothelial surfaces causes mechanical trauma and shear stress.

- Platelet damage.
- Red blood cell hemolysis.

Platelet count is decreased.
Free hemoglobin and hemoglobinuria are increased.
Hct is decreased.

- Leukocyte damage.

Immune response is diminished.

Microembolization

Emboli from tissue debris, air bubbles, platelet aggregation.

Microemboli to body organs (brain, lungs, kidney) are possible.

(continued)

Effects of Cardiopulmonary Bypass (continued)

Causes	Clinical Implications
Increased Systemic Vascular Resistance (SVR)	
Catecholamine secretion increased when cardiopulmonary bypass initiated.	Hypertension is possible. Increased SVR may decrease cardiac output.
Renin secretion due to nonpulsatile flow to kidney.	
Hypothermia.	
Alteration in Carbohydrate Metabolism	
Insulin release is suppressed.	Postoperative hyperglycemia.
Glycogenolysis is stimulated by increase in catecholamines.	Glucosuria may occur.
Decreased perfusion pressure alters glucose transport across cell membrane.	

Complications Associated With PBV

- Embolization of calcific debris
- Valve ring disruption
- Valvular regurgitation
- Valvular restenosis
- Bleeding at arterial puncture site
- Left ventricular perforation
- Severe hypotension
- Transient ischemia
- Vascular trauma
- Atrial septal defect (with mitral PBV)
- Aortic dissection
- Aortic rupture
- Cardiac tamponade
- Chordae tendineae rupture

The Denervated Heart

Effects of Denervation	Implications for Nursing
Resting sinus rate is >90 beats/min.	Slower heart rate can indicate sinus node dysfunction.
Change in heart rate in response to metabolic demands is slower than normal.	Do not use tachycardia as a reliable early sign of decreased cardiac output.
	Instruct patient to warm up and cool down during exercise over 20-min period.
Absence of reflex tachycardia in response to position change and pooling of blood in the extremities can cause orthostatic hypotension.	Instruct patient to change position gradually to prevent dizziness or syncope.
Response to medications whose effects are mediated by the autonomic nervous system is altered.	Treat bradyarrhythmias with isoproterenol or pacing rather than atropine.
	Treat supraventricular tachyarrhythmias with β-blockers, Ca^+ blockers, or cardioversion rather than Valsalva's maneuver, carotid sinus pressure, or digitalis preparations.
	Use isoproterenol, dobutamine, inocor, or epinephrine for inotropic support.
Only mechanism by which heart rate and contractility can increase is through circulating catecholamines.	Use β-blockers with caution.
Transmission of pain impulses from ischemic myocardium is lost.	Patient may have ischemic myocardium but usually does not experience angina.

CHAPTER 4
The Respiratory System

Airway Management

Chest Tubes

Ventilators

COPD and ARDS

Pulmonary Drugs

Checklist of Abnormal Respiratory Findings

Bronchitis

Increased respiratory rate (occasional)

Use of accessory muscles (occasional)

Intercostal retraction (occasional)

Prolonged expiratory phase (frequent)

Increased AP diameter of the chest (frequent)

Decreased motion of the diaphragm (frequent)

Decreased intensity of breath sounds

Crackles

Wheezes (frequent)

Crackles and wheezes clear after cough (frequent)

Pneumothorax

Increased respiratory rate

Trachea deviated to side of pneumothorax

Cyanosis (occasional)

Decreased movement of chest on side of pneumothorax (splint-ing)

Hyperresonance (unreliable sign)

Decreased breath sounds

Decreased tactile fremitus and decreased vocal fremitus (the most reliable signs)

Emphysema

Increased respiratory rate (frequent)

Use of accessory muscles (neck)

Atelectasis

Increased respiratory rate

Increased pulse

Cyanosis (frequent)

Trachea deviated to side of atelectasis

Decreased chest expansion on side of atelectasis (splinting)

Decreased fremitus (tactile and vocal)

Dull or flat percussion note

Decreased breath sounds

Rales (occasional)

Pleural Effusion

Increase in respiratory rate (occasional)

Trachea deviated away from side of effusion

(continued)

Checklist of Abnormal Respiratory Findings (continued)

Decreased fremitus (tactile and vocal)

Decreased breath sounds

Above effusion

Bronchial breathing ⎫
E to A changes ⎬ due to compressed lungs with open airway
Whispered pectoriloquy ⎭

Friction rub—after fluid is removed and visceral pleura rubs against parietal pleura

Decreased intensity (loudness) of breath sounds

Little or no increase in loudness of breath sounds with deep breath

Crackles (frequent)

Wheeze (occasional)

Pneumonia

Increased respiratory rate

Cyanosis (occasional)

Decreased expansion (splinting) (frequent)

Increased fremitus (tactile and vocal)

Palpable rhonchi—usually are removed by coughing or suctioning (occasional)

Dullness to percussion

Bronchial breathing, whispered pectoriloquy, and E to A changes (usual if consolidation is extensive)

Crackles—usually clear with cough or suctioning (occasional)

Pleural friction rub (occasional)

Bronchial breathing, E to A changes, and whispered pectoriloquy if airway is open

Pleural friction rub (occasional)

Large Mass Lesion (tumor)

Dullness over tumor

Fine rales (frequent)

Decreased breath sounds if airway is occluded

Intercostal retractions

Propped up on outstretched arms

Prolonged expiratory phase

Increased AP diameter

Decreased chest expansion

Decreased motion of diaphragm

Hyperresonance to percussion

Subcutaneous Emphysema

Crackling sounds that come from air outside the chest in the soft tissue

Pulmonary Edema (congestive heart failure)

Increased respiratory rate

Cyanosis (frequent)

Use of accessory muscles (usual)

Apprehension

Sitting upright (frequent)

Increased fremitus (due to interstitial edema)

Dull percussion note (due to interstitial edema)

Bronchovesicular sounds (due to interstitial edema, often obscured later by rales)

Crackles that increase in amount, volume, and auscultated area (occasional)

Wheezing (occasional)

Pulmonary Interstitial Fibrosis

Increased respiratory rate (frequent)

Intercostal retractions

Cyanosis (late)

Crackles

Bronchovesicular breathing (occasional)

Body Systems and Possible Events Leading to Respiratory Failure

Systems	Events
1. Nervous system	Head trauma
Brain stem	Poliomyelitis
Spinal cord and nerves	Cervical (C1–C6) fractures
	Overdose
2. Muscular system	Myasthenia gravis
Primary—diaphragm	Guillain–Barré
Secondary—respiratory	
3. Skeletal system	Flail chest
Thorax	Kyphoscoliosis
4. Respiratory system	Obstruction
Airways	Laryngeal edema
	Bronchitis
	Asthma
Alveoli	Emphysema
	Pneumonia
	Fibrosis
Pulmonary circulation	Pulmonary embolus
5. Cardiovascular system	Congestive heart failure
	Fluid overload
	Cardiac surgery
	Myocardial infarction
6. Gastrointestinal system	Aspiration
7. Hematological system	Disseminated intravascular coagulation
8. Genitourinary system	Renal failure

Bedside Measurements of Respiratory Function

Physical Examination

Subjective information (what patient says/writes)

Objective information (what nurse observes)
Daily weight
Urine output/specific gravity
Vital signs
CNS: mental acuity, behavior
Mouth: color of mucosa → ? central cyanosis
Neck: ? prominent neck veins; ? supple
Cardiopulmonary: heart sounds, breath sounds
Abdomen: tenderness or distention?
Extremities: ? cyanosis or clubbing

Pt/Ventilator

Tidal volume (V_T)
Minute ventilation ($\dot{V}_E$)
Inspiratory pressure
Compliance (C_L)

Laboratory

CXR
ECG
ABG
Hgb/Hct
Albumin/Total protein
WBC
Electrolytes

Normal Blood Gas Values

	Arterial Blood	Mixed Venous Blood
pH	7.40 (7.35–7.45)	7.38 (7.33–7.43)
PO_2	80–100 mm Hg	35–49 mm Hg
O_2 sat	95% or greater	70%–75%
PCO_2	35–45 mm Hg	41–51 mm Hg
HCO_3^-	22–26 mEq/L	24–28 mEq/L
Base excess (BE)	−2 to +2	0 to +4

Comparison of PO_2 at Sea Level With PO_2 above Sea Level (>5,000 ft)

At Sea Level	At Denver	Remarks
760	630 mm Hg	Average barometric pressure
−47	−47 mm Hg	Water vapor pressure at body temperature (subtracted because in the body this pressure is exerted by water vapor)
713	583 mm Hg	Corrected barometric pressure (in body or completely humidified air at body temperature)
×21%	×21%	Percent of O_2 in the atmosphere
150 mm Hg	123 mm Hg	PO_2 in air that is completely humidified
−40	−36	PCO_2—pressure exerted by CO_2 in alveolus
110 mm Hg	87 mm Hg	PO_2 in alveolus
−5 mm Hg	−5 mm Hg	Gradient for diffusion of O_2 from alveolus into capillary
105 mm Hg	82 mm Hg	PO_2 in capillary blood in lungs
−10 mm Hg	−10 mm Hg	Due to venous shunting
95 mm Hg	72 mm Hg	PO_2 in arterial blood

Oxygen Values Above Sea Level vs. Sea Level

	Denver	Sea Level
Arterial Blood O_2		
Oxygen content.......	18.9 ml O_2/100 ml of blood	19.7 ml O_2/100 ml of blood
PO_2 .... ∴	70 mm Hg (range 65–75)	>80 mm Hg
O_2 saturation of Hgb ..	93% (range 92%–94%)	≥95%
Mixed Venous Blood O_2		
Oxygen content.......	14–16 ml O_2/100 ml of blood	14–16 ml O_2/100 ml of blood
PO_2	35–49 mm Hg	35–49 mm Hg
O_2 saturation of Hgb ..	70–75%	70–75%
Ratios and Gradients		
a/A ratio............	>.75	>.75
A–a oxygen gradient...	<20	<20

Procedure for Drawing Blood for Arterial Blood Gas Analysis

A. Equipment

1. 5- or 10-ml glass syringe or plastic syringe with vented plunger
2. 10-ml bottle of heparin, 1000 units/ml (multi-dose)
3. No. 22 needle or no. 25 disposable needle (short bevel)
4. Rubber airtight cap
5. Alcohol swab
6. Container of ice (emesis basin or plastic bag)
7. Request slip on which to write patient's clinical status, etc., including
   a. Name, date, time
   b. Whether receiving O_2, and if so show how much and by what route
   c. Temperature

B. Technique

1. Radial artery is generally preferred, although brachial may be used.
2. If a radial approach is used, perform an Allen's test. Simultaneously occlude the radial and ulnar arterial flow. The hand will blanch to pale. Release the ulnar artery flow. A positive Allen's test will return the hand to pink. This ensures arterial flow if the radial artery is no longer patent.
3. Wrist is hyperextended and arm is externally rotated.
   a. Very important to have wrist hyperextended—usually a folded towel under the wrist accomplishes this.
   b. For brachial artery puncture, elbow is hyperextended after placing elbow on towels.
4. 1 ml of heparin is aspirated into the syringe, barrel of the syringe is wet with heparin, and then excess heparin is discarded through the needle, with care taken so that the hub of the needle is left full of heparin and there are no bubbles.
5. Brachial or radial artery is located by palpation with index and long fingers, and point of maximum impulse is found. Clean the site with alcohol.
6. Needle is slowly inserted into the area of maximal pulsation. This is easiest with the syringe and needle approximately 45–90° to the skin.
7. Often the needle goes completely through both sides of the artery and only when the needle is slowly withdrawn does the blood gush up into the syringe.

(continued)

Procedure for Drawing Blood for Arterial Blood Gas Analysis (continued)

8. The only certain indication that arterial blood is obtained is pumping of the blood up into the syringe under its own power.

   a. If one has to aspirate blood by pulling on the plunger of syringe—as is sometimes required with a tighter fitting plastic syringe—it is impossible to be positive that blood is arterial. *The blood gas results do not allow one to determine whether blood is arterial or venous.*

9. After 5 ml of blood are obtained, the needle is withdrawn and the assistant puts constant pressure on site of arterial puncture for at least 5 min (10 min if patient is anticoagulated).

10. Any air bubbles should be squirted out of the syringe. Remove the needle and place airtight rubber stopper on syringe. Roll the syringe between palms to mix the heparin.

11. The syringe is labeled and immediately placed into ice or ice water, then taken to the laboratory.

12. Note:

   a. If O_2 saturation is also measured, this provides a cross-check for accuracy of the PO_2 (use PO_2 and pH to calculate O_2 saturation on blood gas slide rule and see whether this calculated O_2 saturation agrees with the measured O_2 saturation plus carboxyhemoglobin (calculated O_2 saturation = measured O_2 saturation + carboxyhemoglobin).

   b. If CO_2 content is also measured, this provides a cross-check for accuracy of PCO_2. (Use PCO_2 and pH to calculate CO_2 content on blood gas slide rule and see whether this calculated CO_2 content agrees with the measured CO_2 content.)

   c. Another way to ensure accuracy is to run the tests in duplicate on two different blood gas analyzers. If there is a discrepancy in the two determinations, the test must be run a third time.

   d. The technician performing analysis should report any suspicion that results are not reliable. For instance:

      1) If syringe comes with air bubbles in it.

      2) If calculated O_2 saturation and measured O_2 saturation do not agree.

      3) If calculated CO_2 content and measured CO_2 content do not agree.

PCO$_2$, The Respiratory Parameter

PCO_2 = pressure (tension) of dissolved CO_2 gas in blood; influenced only by respiratory causes

Food $\xrightarrow[\text{by body}]{\text{converted}}$ H_2O + CO_2 + energy

CO_2 + $H_2O \rightleftharpoons H_2CO_3 \rightleftharpoons HCO_3^-$ + H^+
Normal PCO_2 = normal ventilation
High PCO_2 = hypoventilation
Low PCO_2 = hyperventilation

Respiratory Abnormalities

Parameter	Condition	Mechanism
↑ PCO_2	Respiratory acidosis	Decreased elimination by lungs of CO_2 gas (hypoventilation)
↓ PCO_2	Respiratory alkalosis	Increased elimination by lungs of CO_2 gas (hyperventilation)

Metabolic Abnormalities

Parameter	Condition	Mechanism
↑ HCO_3^- or ↑ BE	Nonrespiratory (metabolic) alkalosis	1. Nonvolatile acid is lost; or 2. HCO_3^- is gained
↓ HCO_3^- or ↓ BE	Nonrespiratory (metabolic) acidosis	1. Nonvolatile acid is added (using up HCO_3^-); or 2. HCO_3^- is lost

Causes of Respiratory Alkalosis (↓ PCO₂)

Hypoxia

Nervousness and anxiety

Pulmonary embolus, fibrosis, etc.

Pregnancy

Hyperventilation with mechanical ventilator

Brain injury

Salicylates

Fever

Gram-negative septicemia

Hepatic insufficiency

Congestive heart failure

Asthma

Severe anemia

Causes of Respiratory Acidosis (↑ PCO₂)

- Obstructive lung disease
- Oversedation and other causes of reduced function of the respiratory center (even with normal lungs)
- Neuromuscular disorders
- Hypoventilation with mechanical ventilator
- Other causes of hypoventilation: pain, chest wall deformities, etc.

Causes of Metabolic (Nonrespiratory) Alkalosis (↑ HCO₃⁻)

Fluid losses from upper GI tract—vomiting or nasogastric tube causing loss of acid

Rapid correction of chronic hypercapnia

Diuretic therapy—mercurial, ethacrynic acid (Edecrin), furosemide (Lasix), thiazides

Cushing's disease

Therapy with corticosteroids (prednisone, cortisone, etc)

Hyperaldosteronism

Severe potassium depletion

Excessive ingestion of licorice

Bartter's syndrome

Alkali administration

Nonparathyroid hypercalcemia

Causes of Metabolic Acidosis (↓ HCO_3^- and ↓ BE)

Anion Gap:
With Increase in Unspecified
Anions
    Diabetic ketoacidosis
    Starvation ketoacidosis
    Alcoholic ketoacidosis
    Poisonings
        Salicylate
        Ethylene glycol
        Methyl alcohol
        Paraldehyde (rarely)
    Lactic acidosis
    Renal failure

Non-anion Gap:
Without Increase in Unspecified
Anions
    Diarrhea
    Drainage of pancreatic juice
    Ureterosigmoidostomy
    Obstructed ileal loop
    Therapy with acetazolamide
    (Diamox)
    Therapy with ammonium chloride (NH_4Cl)
    Renal tubular acidosis
    Intravenous hyperalimentation
    (rarely)
    Dilutional acidosis

Compensation Versus Correction of Acid–Base Abnormalities

In both: Abnormal pH is returned toward normal.

    Compensation: Abnormal pH is returned toward normal *by altering the component not primarily affected;* that is, if PCO_2 is high, HCO_3^- is retained to compensate.

    Correction: Abnormal pH is returned toward normal *by altering the component primarily affected;* that is, if PCO_2 is high, PCO_2 is lowered, correcting the abnormality.

Signs and Symptoms of Acid–Base Disorders

Acid–Base Disorder	Signs & Symptoms
Respiratory Acidosis	Signs of CO_2 narcosis: headache lethargy drowsiness coma increased heart rate hypertension sweating decreased responsiveness tremulousness/asterixis papilledema dyspnea (may or may not be present)
Respiratory Alkalosis	Vague symptoms: dizziness numbness tingling (parasthesia) of the extremities muscle cramps tetany seizures increases in deep tendon reflexes arrhythmias hyperventilation
Metabolic Acidosis	Kussmaul breathing Hypotension Lethargy Nausea and vomiting
Metabolic Alkalosis	Nonspecific: hyperactive reflexes tetany hypertension muscle cramps weakness

Compensation for Acidosis and Alkalosis

Parameter	Normal	Abnormal* (Uncompensated)	Compensated
Respiratory Acidosis			
HCO_3^- mEq/L	24	24	36
PCO_2 mEq/L	1.2	1.8	1.8
PCO_2 mm HG	40	60	60
ratio	20:1	13:1	20:1
pH	7.40	7.23	7.40
Respiratory Alkalosis			
BE	0	+2.5	−5
HCO_3^- mEq/L	24	24	18
PCO_2 mEq/L	1.2	0.9	0.9
PCO_2 mm Hg	40	30	30
ratio	20:1	27:1	20:1
pH	7.40	7.52	7.40
Metabolic Acidosis			
BE	0	−17	−10
HCO_3^- mEq/L	24	12	12
PCO_2 mEq/L	1.2	1.2	0.6
PCO_2 mm Hg	40	40	20
ratio	20:1	10:1	20:1
pH	7.40	7.11	7.40
Metabolic Alkalosis			
BE	0	+13	+9
HCO_3^- mEq/L	24	36	36
PCO_2 mEq/L	1.2	1.2	1.8
PCO_2 mm Hg	40	40	60
ratio	20:1	30:1	20:1
pH	7.40	7.57	7.40

*The primary abnormality is in the enclosed box.

Contraindications for Chest Physiotherapy

Postural Drainage	Percussion	Vibration
Increased intracranial pressure	Fractured ribs	Same as percussion
Immediately after meals	Traumatic chest injury	
Inability to cough	Pulmonary hemorrhage or embolus	
Acute heart disease	Mastectomy	
Intravascular bleeds	Orthopedic appliances	
	Pneumothorax	
	Metastatic lesion of ribs	
	Osteoporosis	
	Cervical cord trauma	
	Unstable fractures	
	Abdominal trauma	
	Hiatal hernia	
	Obesity	

IPPB (Intermittent Positive Pressure Breathing)

Indications	Contraindications
Reduced vital capacity	Pneumothorax
Failure of simpler methods such as postural drainage and coughing, deep breathing and coughing, incentive spirometry, and hydration to expel secretions	Bullous emphysema
	Increased intracranial pressure
	Tracheoesophageal fistula
	Bronchopleural fistula
Restrictive disorders (ascites, interstitial disease, kyphoscoliosis)	Hypovolemia
	Increased dyspnea during treatment
Pulmonary edema	Hemoptysis
Neuromuscular deficits	Immediately after lung resection; pneumonectomy
Sputum induction for tests	Active pulmonary TB
Medication delivery (especially in patients with severe hand deformities)	Gastric reflux condition (tube feedings or meals within the last hour)

Airway Placement

Type	Advantages	Disadvantages
Nasal endotracheal	Patient comfort	Can kink and obstruct the airway
	Prevents tube obstruction from biting	Predisposes to nasal or sinus infection
	Easily anchored	Tube and cuff can cause tracheal damage
		High risk for shearing off nasal polyps in asthmatics
Oral endotracheal	Less trauma during intubation than nasally	Predisposes to mouth sores
	Permits use of a larger ET tube	Uncomfortable for patient
		Easily obstructed if not used with bite block
		Tube and cuff can cause tracheal damage
		Complicates effective oral hygiene
		Difficult to secure

Complications of Tracheal Intubation

Trauma
Nosocomial infection
Mechanical problems
Displacement of Tube:
• right mainstem intubation
• gastric intubation
Aspiration
Physiologic problems (tracheal necrosis)
Laryngeal damage and necrosis

Endotracheal Tube Sizes

Patient	ET Tube Size	Suction Catheter
Adult Female	7.0 mm	10 FR
	8.0 mm	12 FR
	8.5 mm	14 FR
Adult Male	8.5 mm	14 FR
	9.0 mm	16 FR
	10.0 mm	18 FR

Early Conversion From ET Tube to Tracheostomy Tube

Advantages	Disadvantages
Prevents further injury from ET tube	Cost of procedure
Increases patient comfort and psychological well-being	Risk of bleeding
	Risk of dislodging tube into SQ tissues
Facilitates suctioning and mouth care	Scar and/or disfigurement
More secure artificial airway	
Facilitates ambulation and allows for transfer to non-acute setting	
Permits verbal communication	
Facilitates oral nourishment	

Indication for Chest Tube Placement

Indication	Cause
Hemothorax	Chest trauma
	Neoplasms
	Pleural tears
	Excessive anticoagulation
	Post thoracic surgery
Pneumothorax	
Spontaneous: >20%	Bleb rupture
Symptomatic patient	
Presence of lung disease	
Tension	Mechanical ventilation
	Penetrating puncture wound
	Prolonged clamping of chest tubes
	Lack of seal in chest tube drainage system
Bronchopleural fistula	Tissue damage
	Tumor
	Aspiration of toxic chemicals
Pleural Effusion	Neoplasms
Complicated parapneumonia:	Serious cardiopulmonary disease
Gross pus (empyema)	Inflammatory conditions
Gram-positive stain or bacterial culture	
Glucose <40 mg/dl	
pH <7.0	
pH 7.0–7.2 and LDH >1000 IU/L	
Chylothorax	Trauma
	Malignancy
	Congenital abnormalities

Chest Tube Drainage Systems

System	Advantages	Disadvantages
One-Bottle	Simple configuration Easy to ambulate patient	As chest drainage fills up the bottle, more force is needed to allow pleural air and liquid to exit the chest into the bottle A mixture of drained blood and air creates a frothy mixture in the bottle that limits precise measurement of drainage To drain, pleural pressures must be higher than bottle pressures
Two-Bottle	Keeps the water seal at a constant level Allows better observation and measurement of drainage	Adds dead space to the drainage system that has the potential to be drawn into the pleural space To drain, pleural pressures must be higher than bottle pressures Has limitations on excessive air flow capacity in presence of a pleural leak
Three-Bottle	Safest system to regulate suction	More complex, more room for error in the set up and in maintenance
Disposable Units Water seal	Plastic and do not break as easily as bottles	Cost Loss of water seal and accuracy of drainage measurement if unit is tipped over
Flutter valve	Ideal for transport since water seal is maintained if unit tips over One less chamber to fill No problems with evaporation of water Decreased noise level	Cost Valve device doesn't provide visual information on intrapleural pressures because of absence of water fluctuations in the water seal chamber

Screw-valve	Same as above	Narrow valve limits the amount of volume it can handle; inefficient for large pleural air leaks
Calibrated spring mechanism	Same as above Able to handle large volumes	Cost

---

Signs and Symptoms of Tension Pneumothorax

- Tachycardia
- Tachypnea
- Agitation
- Diaphoresis
- Midline tracheal shift
- Muffled heart tones
- Absent breath sounds over affected lung

- Hyper-resonance to percussion over affected lung
- Hypotension
- Cardiac arrest
- High pressure alarms (if mechanically ventilated)

Underwater Seal Drainage Systems

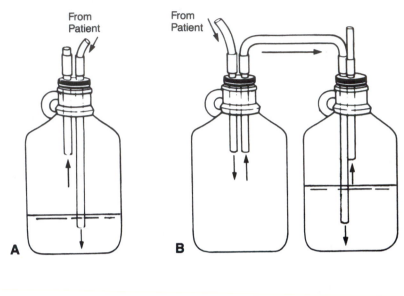

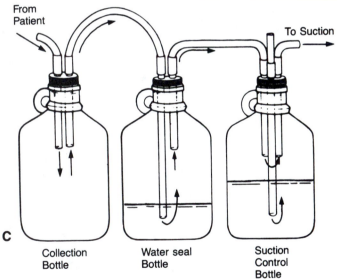

Collection Bottle

Water seal Bottle

Suction Control Bottle

(A) One-bottle system underwater seal drainage. (B) Two-bottle system underwater seal drainage. (C) Underwater seal drainage with suction.

Potential Complications of Chest Tube Stripping

Generation of excessive negative pressures causing aspiration of lung tissue into eyelets of chest tube

Rupture of alveoli

Persistent pleural leak

Disrupted suture lines

Acute myocardial ischemia

Increase in pulmonary wedge pressure

Increase in venous return to the right heart

Shift in the ventricular septum to the left

Right ventricular interference with left ventricular function

Impedance to left ventricular ejection

Indications for Chest Tube Removal

- One day after cessation of air leak
- Drainage of <50–100 cc of fluid per day
- 1–3 days post cardiac surgery
- 2–6 days post thoracic surgery
- Obliteration of empyema cavity
- Serosanguinous drainage from around the chest tube insertion site

Indications for Mechanical Ventilation

Parameters	Values	Action
Respiratory rate	<10 breaths/min (diminished drive to breathe)	Evaluate patient and eliminate cause
	16–20 breaths/min	Normal
	28–40 breaths/min	Evaluate patient and institute appropriate measures
	>40 breaths/min	Consider elective intubation/ventilation
Vital capacity	<10–20 ml/kg (poor ventilatory reserve)	Watch for signs of respiratory failure
		Prepare to initiate ventilatory support
Inspiratory pressures	<20 cm water or decreasing trend	
Arterial blood gases		
pH	<7.25	Evaluate in combination with rising $PaCO_2$
$PaCO_2$	>50 mm Hg	Evaluate in combination with decreasing pH
PaO_2	<50 mm Hg while on O_2	Evaluate in combination with the pH and $PaCO_2$
A – a gradient Shunt	≥300 mm Hg	
	≥25–30	
Chest auscultation	Diminished or no breath sounds	Deliver 100% O_2
		Prepare ventilatory support
Heart rate and rhythm	Pulse over 120, dysrhythmias	Monitor for dysrhythmias
Activity	Extreme fatigue, lessened activity tolerance	Evaluate with above and take appropriate measures
Mental status	Confusion, delirium, somnolence	Monitor for hypoxic seizure activity
Physical observation	Use of accessory muscles, fatiguing, extreme work of breathing	Prepare for ventilatory support

Complications of Mechanical Ventilation

Airway

Aspiration

Decreased clearance of secretions

Predisposition to infection

Endotracheal Tube

Tube kinked

Tube plugged

Rupture of pyriform sinus

Tracheal stenosis

Tracheal malacia

Right main stem intubation

Cuff failure

Sinusitis

Otitis media

Laryngeal edema

Mechanical

Ventilator malfunction

Hypoventilation

Hyperventilation

Tension pneumothorax

Physiological

Water and NaCl retention

Left ventricular dysfunction →
hypotension

Stress ulcers

Paralytic ileus

Gastric distention

Starvation

Hyperinflation and Hyperoxygenation Prior to Suctioning

Method	Advantages	Disadvantages
Manual resuscitator bag	Ability to feel lung compliance	Requires ventilator disconnection which affects oxygen saturation and PEEP levels
	Ability to vary flows and volumes to remove mucous plugs	
		Inconsistent delivery of volumes and oxygen
		Generates unknown airway pressures
Ventilator	Maintenance of PEEP levels	Easy to forget to return setting to previous level
	Fewer effects on hemodynamics	Requires a "washout period" for oxygen to reach 100% delivered

Criteria for Weaning

Weaning Tests

Vital Capacity (VC): 10–15 cc/kg

Tidal Volume (V$_T$): 4–5 cc/kg

Minute Ventilation (MV):* 6–10 liters

Maximum Voluntary Ventilation (MVV)†: Double the MV

Inspiratory Force‡: 20 cm H$_2$O or greater

Compliance: −20 ml/cm H$_2$O or greater

RR: <20/min

Ventilator Settings

FIO$_2$: <.50

PEEP: 0

V$_T$: Average for the patient

ABGs

PaCO$_2$: Normal for the patient

P(A − a)O$_2$: >200–300 mm Hg (100% FIO$_2$)

PaO$_2$: 60-mid 70 or normal for patient

pH: Normal with all electrolyte imbalances corrected

Endotracheal Tube

Position: Above the carina on x-ray

Size: 8.5 mm diameter or greater

Tracheostomy: For long-term weans

Nutrition

Daily calories: 2000–2500/day

Day of wean: 1000 with limited glucose intake

Time: At least 1 h after a meal

Airway

Secretions: Antibiotics if change in color; suctioned well and rested

Bronchospasms: Controlled with β-adrenergics, theophyllines, or steroids

Position: Up in chair, semi-Fowler's, or positioned for maximizing air exchange or diaphragm movement

Drugs

Sedating agents: Stopped more than 24 h

Paralyzing agents: Stopped more than 24 h

(*continued*)

Criteria for Weaning (continued)

Emotional

"Psyched up" for the wean

Physical

Stable; no new acute process; rested

---

* Minute Ventilation. If MV is higher than 20 liters, the work of breathing is high. The patient may well wean, but after a couple of hours may fatigue and need to be reintubated. When MV is less than 6 liters, hypoventilation will occur. The etiology for hypoventilation needs to be investigated because often the cause is sedation.

† Maximum Voluntary Ventilation (MVV) is obtained by having the patient breathe as hard and as fast as possible for 15 sec. Multiply this by 4 and the answer is total MVV for 1 min. MVV is an objective measurement of the patient's ventilatory reserve. If the patient's work of breathing postextubation is increased and ventilatory reserve is low, reintubation may be needed.

‡ Inspiratory Pressure. Inspiratory pressure gives an indication of inspiratory muscle strength. A pressure less than -20 ml/cm H_2O pressure indicates muscle weakness. The work of breathing will be very costly and fatigue will result.

Adjuncts to Weaning

Fenestrated Trach*

- Provides for communication during weaning periods

Kirshner Button

- Provides for communication during weaning periods
- Less resistance to breathing and coughing up secretions than with the fenestrated trach

Large ET Tubes (>8.5 mm)

- Small-diameter endotracheal tubes increase resistance to breathing, thereby increasing work of breathing

Postural Drainage and Percussion

- Aids in removal of secretions

Exercise

- Provides increased stimulation to breathing
- Increases and changes environmental stimuli

Nutrition

- Provides energy for breathing
- Maintains protein balance
- Aids in resistance to infection

IPPB

- Provides periods of hyperinflation and rest during weaning periods
- May maintain patient when weaned

Pulse Oximetry

- Provides noninvasive monitoring of O_2 saturation

---

* The fenestrated trach tube has an opening in the outer cannula but not the inner cannula. With the inner cannula in place and the cuff inflated, the patient is easily mechanically ventilated. During the weaning process, the inner cannula is removed, the cuff deflated, the outer cannula capped, and supplemental oxygen supplied via nasal cannula. This system permits air to pass from the patient's nares through the hole in the outer cannula (fenestration in the trach tube) and past the vocal cords, allowing verbal communication on the part of the patient.

Assessment Criteria That May Terminate Weaning From Mechanical Ventilation

Physiological Data

Pulse: Increase or decrease of 20 beats/min or more

Blood pressure: Systolic increase or decrease of 20 mm Hg

Respiratory rate: Change of 10 breaths/min; respiratory rate >25 breaths/min or <8 breaths/min

Psychological/Subjective Data

Dyspnea

Panic

Pain

Fatigue

Objective Observations

Dysrhythmias: PVCs >4/min

Increased accessory muscle use

Increased intercostal retractions

Increased flaring of nostrils

Erratic breathing pattern (paradoxical breathing, increased restlessness, increased drowsiness)

ABGs deteriorating: Increased $PaCO_2$ resulting in pH < 7.35 or oxygen desaturation via oximetry

Troubleshooting the Ventilator

Problem	Possible Causes	Action
Volume or pressure alarm on	*Patient-Related*	
	Patient disconnected from ventilator	Reconnect stat.
	Loss of delivered V_T	Occlude endotracheal tube adaptor—if alarm goes off, there is a patient problem; if not, there is a ventilator problem
		Auscultate neck for possible leak around ET cuff
		Review chest film for endotracheal tube placement—may be too high
		Check for loss of V_T through chest tube
	Decrease in patient-initiated breaths	Evaluate patient for cause: check respiratory rate, ABGs, last sedation dosage
	Increased compliance	Good news! May be due to clearing of secretions or relief of bronchospasms
	Ventilator-Related	
	Leaks	Check all tubing for loss of connection, starting at patient and moving toward the ventilator
		Tighten cascade humidifier
		Determine whether ventilator settings have changed
		Check for interference with spirometer dipstick
		Calibrate spirometer or pressure alarm
		If all else fails, replace exhalation valve (*Note:* If problem is not corrected stat, bag-breathe patient until respirator problem is corrected)

High-pressure or peak-pressure alarm	Decreased pressure to ventilator on pressure-driven ventilator (*eg*, Monaghan or Bird)	Have engineering department check pressure line; must deliver 50 psi
	Patient-Related	
	Decreased compliance	
	Increased dynamic pressures	Suction patient
		Administer inhaled β-agonists
		If sudden, evaluate for pneumothorax
		Alleviate coughing with sedation or lidocaine
		Try to change patient's position
		Evaluate chest film for endotracheal tube placement in right main stem bronchus
		Sedate if patient is bucking the ventilator or biting the ET tube
	Increased static pressures	Evaluate ABGs for hypoxia, fluids for overload, chest film for atelectasis
		Auscultate breath sounds
	Ventilator-Related	
	Tubing kinked	Check tubing
	Tubing filled with water	Empty water into a receptacle; do not drain back into the humidifier (*Note:* Water in tubing will increase PEEP levels)
	Patient–ventilator asynchrony	Recheck sensitivity and peak flow settings

(continued)

Troubleshooting the Ventilator *(continued)*

Problem	Possible Causes	Action
Abnormal ABGs	*Patient-Related*	
Hypoxia	Secretions	Suction
	Increase in disease pathology	Evaluate patient and chest film
	Positive fluid balance	Evaluate intake and output
Hypocapnia	Hypoxia	Evaluate ABGs and patient
	Increased lung compliance	Good news; evaluate for weaning potential
Hypercapnia	Sedation	Increase respiratory rate or V_T settings on ventilator
	Fatigue	
	Ventilator-Related	
Hypoxia	F_IO_2 drift	Check ventilator with oxygen analyzer
		Possible blender piping failure
		Check oxygen source for failure
		Check oxygen reservoir for leaks
Hypocapnia	Settings not set correctly	Decrease respiratory rate, V_T, or MV settings. Consider dead space if assist–control is used
Hypercapnia	Settings not set correctly	Increase respiratory rate, V_T, or MV settings
Heater alarm	Addition of cool water to humidifier	Wait
	Altered setting	Reset
	Faulty temperature gauge	Replace gauge
	Thermostat failure	Replace heater

Manifestations of Severe Exacerbations of Chronic Bronchitis

Constitutional Signs

Temperature frequently subnormal
  WBC varies—may be slightly
  ↑, normal, or ↓

CNS Disturbances

Headache
Confusion
Hallucinations
Depression
Drowsiness
Somnolence
Coma
Papilledema

Cardiovascular Signs

Diaphoresis
Tachycardia
Blood pressure varies:
  Normal, ↑, or ↓
  Vasoconstriction initially followed by vasodilation

Neuromuscular Signs

Fine tremors
Asterixis
Flaccidity
Convulsions

COPD: *Features That Distinguish Bronchitis and Emphysema*

Features	Bronchitis	Emphysema
Primary Location of Pathology	Airways	Air sacs
Clinical Examination		
Subjective Data	Frequent recurrent chest infections	Frequently only insidious dyspnea—initially with exercise only, then progressing
	Sputum production	
	Cough	
Objective Data		
Appearance	"Blue bloaters"	"Pink puffers"
Chest examination	Noisy chest, *slight* overdistention	Quiet chest, marked overdistention
Sputum	Frequently copious and purulent	Usually scant and mucoid
Chronic cor pulmonale	Common—may occur relatively early	Infrequent until terminal stages
Laboratory Tests		
ABGs		
Chronic hypoxemia	Often significant	Usually mild
Chronic hypercapnia	Common	Uncommon
Spirometry		
FEV_1/FVC	Decreased	Decreased
FEV_1	Decreased	Decreased
Therapeutic Modalities		
Bronchial hygiene (measures to enhance secretion clearance)	Very important	Less important unless patient has respiratory infection

Summary: Interstitial Lung Disease

I. *Pathology of ILD*
   A. Primary process—active inflammation (alveolitis)
   B. Secondary process—fibrosis

II. *Pathophysiology*
   A. Alveolitis involving lymphocytes—exposure to an antigen is the initiating event
   B. Alveolitis involving neutrophils—production of chemical mediators potentially toxic to components of alveolar walls

III. *Pathophysiology basic to majority of ILD*
   Inflammation and fibrosis of alveolar wall components:
   A. Decreased pulmonary compliance (increased stiffness) due to significant inflammatory and fibrotic process
   B. Generalized decrease in lung volume due to change in compliance (stiffness) of the lung
   C. Impaired diffusion of O_2 and CO_2 due to destruction of alveolar–capillary walls with resultant decrease of available surface area for gas exchange
   D. Disturbances in gas exchange (primarily ↓ PaO_2) secondary to disruption of normal matching of ventilation and perfusion

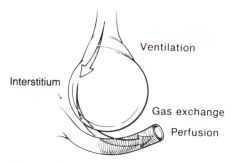

   E. Pulmonary hypertension—ultimate sequelae with severe ILD secondary to:
      (1) bronchoconstriction associated with hypoxemia and
      (2) destruction of small pulmonary vessels by the alveolar wall fibrotic process

IV. *Clinical features/assessment*
   A. Dyspnea on exertion progressing to dyspnea at rest
   B. Cough—usually nonproductive
   C. Velcro (dry) crackles—most prominent at base of lungs

V. *Diagnosis*
   A. Chest roentgenogram
   B. Bronchoscopy/biopsy/lavage—as indicated
   C. Open lung biopsy—as indicated/appropriate

VI. *Management*
   A. Corticosteroids— ↓ inflammatory process
   B. Immunosuppressive agents—eg, Imuran

Signs and Symptoms of Sleep Apnea

Daytime drowsiness
Headache on awakening
Intermittent loud snoring
Apnea spells of 10 to 100 sec or longer
Difficulty concentrating
Personality changes

Reduced libido
Restless sleep
Cardiac rhythm disturbances
Pulmonary hypertension
Hypoxemia
Right ventricular failure

Disorders Predisposing to ARDS

Systemic
  Shock, of any etiology
  Gram-negative sepsis
  Hypothermia
  Hyperthermia
  Drug overdose
    Narcotic
    Salicylate
    Tricyclic
    Paraquat
    Methadone
    Bleomycin
  Hematologic disorders
    Disseminated intravascular coagulation
    Massive transfusion
    Cardiopulmonary bypass
  Eclampsia
  Burns

Pulmonary
  Pneumonia
    Viral
    Bacterial
    Fungal
    Pneumocystic carinii
  Trauma
    Fat emboli
    Lung contusion
  Aspiration
    Gastric fluids
    Near-drowning
    Hydrocarbon fluids
  Pneumonitis
Nonpulmonary
  Head injury
  Increased intracranial pressure
  Postcardioversion
  Pancreatitis
  Uremia

ARDS: Summary of Clinical Assessment Through Management Process

A. Precipitating pulmonary or nonpulmonary event
B. Clinical signs/assessment
   1. Tachypnea
   2. Tachycardia
   3. Labored respirations
   4. Use of accessory muscles
C. Laboratory findings
   1. ABG analysis: $\downarrow\downarrow$ PaO_2 (ie, < 50 mm with supplemental O_2)
                   $\downarrow$ $PaCO_2$
   2. Chest radiograph: diffuse bilateral pulmonary infiltrates
   3. High $\dot{V}_E$ (ie, >20 L/min)
   4. Low left atrial pressure via pulmonary artery catheter
D. Management
   1. Establishment of definitive airway: endotracheal tube/tracheostomy
   2. Mechanical ventilation: volume ventilator with high pressure and flow capabilities
   3. PEEP
   4. Monitoring for adequate arterial oxygenation
   5. Fluids
   6. Pharmacological agents (ie, O_2 and diuretics; antibiotics for documented infection)
   7. Airway maintenance
   8. Prevention of infection
   9. Nutritional support
   10. Monitor *all* systems for response to therapy and potential complications
   11. Treatment of underlying condition
E. Prognosis: approximately 50% to 70% mortality
F. Sequelae on recovery: infrequent

Action, Dosage, and Side Effects of Pulmonary Drugs

Pulmonary Drugs	Action	Dosage	Side Effects
1. Broncholidilators			
Methylxanthines	↓ phosphodiesterase with ↑ cyclic AMP (active form)	IV: loading—5 mg/kg; maintenance—0.9 mg/kg PO: aminophylline—1200 mg/24 hr; oxtriphylline (Choledyl)—1600 mg/24 hr NB: Dosages adjusted to maintain serum theophylline levels 10–20 µg/ml	Nausea Vomiting Nervousness Dysrhythmias Seizures

Theophylline—Dosage increased by 50% for smokers who can tolerate the drug if effect is less than optimal. Dosage decreased by 50% for patients with liver failure, heart failure, hypoxemia, and shock.

Sympathomimetics	β-Stimulants		Relatively few side effects with recommended dosages
Isoetharine (Bronkosol)	Stimulates adenyl cyclase with ↑ cyclic AMP (active form)	Delivered by nebulizer—either hand-powered or IPPB 0.5 ml with sterile water or normal saline (1:3 conc.) q4h	Tachycardia Palpitations Nausea Headache Changes in blood pressure Nervousness

Drug	Mechanism	Dose	Side Effects
Terbutaline (Brethine)	Stimulates adenyl cyclase with ↑ cyclic AMP (active form)	5 mg PO q8h; 0.25 mg SC not to exceed 0.5 mg q4h	↑ Heart rate Nervousness Tremor Palpitations Dizziness (Usually transient effects and do not require treatment)
Metaproterenol (Alupent, Metaprel)	Stimulates adenyl cyclase with ↑ cyclic AMP (active form)	Metered dose device: 0.65 mg/metered dose; 20 mg PO tid	Tachycardia Hypertension Palpitations Nervousness Tremor Nausea and vomiting
Albuterol (Salbutamol, Proventyl)	Same as for metaproterenol	Metered dose device: 1–2 inhalations q4–6h Oral: 2–4 mg q6–8h	Mainly fine finger tremors
Bitolterol (Tornolate)	Same as for metaproterenol	Metered dose: 370 mg/puff 2 puffs q4–6h	Derivative of metaproterenol
Fenoterol (Berota)	Same as for metaproterenol	7.5 mg PO bid/tid and corresponding aerosol dose: 400 mg	See metaproterenol

(*continued*)

Action, Dosage, and Side Effects of Pulmonary Drugs (continued)

Pulmonary Drugs	Action	Dosage	Side Effects
Epinephrine	Same as for metaproterenol	0.2–0.5 mg of 1:1000 solution SC q2h as necessary. Severe attacks: doses may be repeated every 20 min for maximum of three doses	Anxiety Tremors Palpitations Tachycardia Hirsutism (Contraindicated in hypertension, hyperthyroidism, ischemic heart disease, and cerebrovascular insufficiency)

Summary of Potential Systemic Effects of Sympathomimetics

Neurological—	Tremulousness, agitation, anxiety, insomnia, dizziness, faintness
Ophthalmic—	Glaucoma
Cardiovascular—	Tachycardia, palpitations, dysrhythmias, alterations in blood pressure, angina, vasodilation or vasoconstriction, myocardial necrosis
Respiratory—	Tracheal and/or bronchial irritation, bronchospasm (paradoxical response), blood gases—decreased PaO_2
Metabolic—	Hyperglycemia, hyperthyroidism
Gastrointestinal—	Nausea, vomiting, dry mouth, gagging
Genitourinary—	Urinary retention—primarily in men with prostate hypertrophy
Interaction with other drugs—	Insulin, oral hypoglycemic agents, monoamine oxidase inhibitors, general anesthetics, hypotensive agents, thyroid hormone

2. Steroids   Stimulate adenylate cyclase with ↑ cyclic 3′, 5′-AMP; may facilitate use of β-stimulants; anti-inflammatory action

Prednisone

Variable; eg, 40–60 mg PO initially and decreasing according to PFT and eosinophil counts (in patients with ↑ Eos 2° to allergin-mediated responses)

Formation of glucose from body protein → ↑ blood sugar

Depletion of bone calcium—osteoporosis

Increase in fat production

Impairment of immunologic response

Reduction of inflammatory response

Increase in gastric acidity

Elevation of blood pressure

Acne

Methylpred-
   nisolone
   (Solu-Medrol)

Variable; eg, 100 mg IV and repeat with one fourth original dose q6h

Same as for prednisone

(continued)

Action, Dosage, and Side Effects of Pulmonary Drugs (continued)

Pulmonary Drugs	Action	Dosage	Side Effects
Beclomethasone (Vanceril)	Virtually same as for other steroids except it is an inhaled preparation with a high topical effect on the airways and low systemic activity	Inhalation device; 2 inhalations (100 μg) qid	Oral candidiasis Mild oropharyngeal symptoms—discomfort and dryness of throat
3. Cromolyn Sodium (Aarane, Intal)	Prophylactic bronchospasmolytic in allergic asthma; *not* useful in acute bronchospasm; probably strengthens mast cell membrane, preventing release of histamine and therefore decreases bronchospasm in the allergic asthmatic	1 capsule via inhaler device qid	Maculopapular rash Urticaria Cough and/or bronchospasm
4. Anticholinergics Atropine sulfate	Parasympathetic antagonist	5 mg of solution	Tachycardia Dry mouth

Antibiotic Therapy in Pulmonary Disease *

Pulmonary Complication	Antibiotic	Dosage
Pneumococcal pneumonia with or without COPD	Penicillin	600,000 U procaine penicillin IM q12h (a blood level of 0.02 mg/ml 12 h after start of drug is adequate to kill organism) or IV prep: aqueous penicillin G 300,000–600,000 U IV q3–4h
	Penicillin V	250 mg orally q6h
	Cefazolin	500 mg IM or IV q8h
	Cephalexin	500 mg orally q6h
Staphylococcus pneumonia (production of enzymes that destroy lung tissue)	Antistaphylococcal agents Nafcillin Methicillin Cloxacillin Penicillin	1–2 g IV q4–6h
Klebsiella pneumonia (gram-negative): a very severe pneumonia with high mortality; seen more commonly in chronic/debilitated states[†]	Cephalosporin (Cefazolin)	1 g IM or IV q4–6h
	Gentamicin	Dosage is related to renal function (ie, creatinine clearance); commonly, 3–6 mg/kg/24 h. Aim to achieve a trough blood level not less than 1.5 mg/ml and a peak level not over 10 mg/ml
Pseudomonas pneumonia (gram-negative)[†]	Tobramycin	3–5 mg/kg/24 h, producing blood levels of 2.5 mg/ml in presence of normal renal function
	Gentamicin	3–5 mg/kg/24 h (see *Klebsiella* pneumonia, above)

(continued)

Antibiotic Therapy in Pulmonary Disease* (continued)

Pulmonary Complication	Antibiotic	Dosage
Haemophilus influenza	Ampicillin	2.0–6.0 g/24 h, increasing to 8–12 g/24 h for serious infections
	Chloramphenicol	3.0–4.0 g/24 h PO (50–100 mg/kg/24 h)

* A complete discussion of antibiotic therapy related to pulmonary disease and/or complications is beyond the scope of this chapter.

† Antibiotic treatment of gram-negative bacterial pneumonias frequently consists of aminoglycoside and a second drug (ie, a cephalosporin). The rationale is based on poor penetration into bronchial secretions by aminoglycosides; in addition, antibiotic resistance occurs frequently with the latter.

CHAPTER 5
The Renal System

Assessment and Diagnosis

Acute Renal Failure

End-Stage Renal Disease and Renal Transplantation

Electrolyte Abnormalities: Sodium

Electrolyte	Abnormality	Assessment Findings	Causes
Sodium	Hypernatremia Na > 145 mEq/L	Sticky or dry oral mucous membranes; thirst; hypotension; firm body tissues; tachycardia, oliguria or anuria, anxiety	• Increased sodium intake or decreased water intake (ie, aldosteronism) • Inhalation of salt water in near drowning • Hypertonic tube feedings • High-dose steroids • Excessive infusion of saline solutions
	Hyponatremia Na < 135 mEq/L 135–125 mEq/L	Generally none	• Increased water intake with decreased sodium intake (ie, diuretics, excess IV D5W, gastric suction [especially with tap water irrigation or ice chip ingestion]) • Vomiting • Diarrhea
	125–110 mEq/L	Headache, apathy, lethargy, weakness, disorientation	• Repeated tap water enemas • Water replacement without salt replacement in a hot environment that causes diaphoresis
	110–100 mEq/L	Confusion, hostility; lethargy or violence; nausea and vomiting; areflexia	• Addison's disease • SIADH that occurs in patient's with CNS disturbances, patients on ventilators, and those with oat cell cancer
	100–95 mEq/L	Delirium, convulsions, coma, hypothermia; Cheyne–Stokes respiration; death	• Excessive beer intake • Inhalation of fresh water in near drowning

D5W, Dextrose 5% in water; SIADH, syndrome of inappropriate antidiuretic hormone secretion; CNS, central nervous system.

Electrolyte Abnormalities: Potassium

Electrolyte	Abnormality	Assessment Findings	Causes
Potassium	Hyperkalemia K > 5.0 mEq/L	Irritability and restlessness; anxiety; nausea, vomiting, and diarrhea; muscle cramps, weakness; paresthesias; ECG changes with cardiac irregularities; peaked T waves, ventricular fibrillation, cardiac arrest	• Renal failure • Excessive K$^+$ replacement • Initial reaction to massive tissue damage (ie, burns, trauma, metabolic acidosis) • Hypoaldosteronism • Potassium-sparing diuretics
	Hypokalemia K < 3.5 mEq/L	Fatigue that progresses to paralysis; paresthesias; nausea, vomiting, anorexia, dizziness; confusion; ventricular ectopy, cardiac arrest; increased sensitivity to digitalis	• Inadequate intake • Vomiting, diarrhea, suctioning, wound drainage • Excessive diaphoresis • Metabolic alkalosis • Hyperaldosteronism • Diuretic phase of renal failure • Insulin drip for DKA

ECG, electrocardiograph; DKA, diabetic ketoacidosis.

Electrolyte Abnormalities: Calcium and Phosphate

Electrolyte	Abnormality	Assessment Findings	Causes
Calcium	Hypercalcemia Ca > 10.5 mg/dl	Muscle weakness/atrophy; lethargy, coma; personality or behavioral changes; pathologic fractures; bone pain; polyuria; excessive thirst; anorexia, nausea, vomiting, constipation; hypertension; ECG changes (ie, shortened QT, AV block)	• Increased intestinal absorption • Excessive vitamin D • Increased bone resorption • Immobility • Thiazide diuretics • Hyperparathyroidism • Multiple fractures • Decreased phosphorus
	Hypocalcemia Ca < 8.5 mg/dl	Paresthesias, tetany, seizures, abdominal spasms, cramps; skeletal muscle cramps; laryngeal spasm; positive Chvostek's and Trousseau's signs, impaired memory, irritability; decreased cardiac output; bleeding	• Renal failure • Protein malnutrition or malabsorption • Decreased intake • Burns or infection • Hypoparathyroidism • Diarrhea • Excessive antacid use • Multiple blood transfusions • Acute pancreatitis • Liver disease • Vitamin D intoxication • Elevated phosphate
Phosphate	Hyperphosphatemia > 4.5 mg/dl	Tachycardia; nausea, diarrhea, abdominal cramps; muscle weakness, paralysis, increased reflexes; decreased calcium	• Renal failure • Hypoparathyroidism • Lactic acidosis • Chemotherapy, certain malignancies • Hypocalcemia, vitamin D intoxication

	Assessment Findings	Causes
Hypophosphatemia < 3 mg/dl	Ataxia, paresthesias, confusion, coma, seizures; muscle weakness, joint stiffness, bone pain; anorexia, dysphagia; anemia, platelet dysfunction, impaired immunity	• Decreased intake or malabsorption • DKA • Excessive antacid use • Lack of vitamin D • Alkalosis, hyperparathyroidism, renal tubule defects • Insulin therapy in DKA, alcoholism

AV, atrioventricular; DKA, diabetic ketoacidosis.

Electrolyte Abnormalities: Magnesium

Electrolyte	Abnormality	Assessment Findings	Causes
Magnesium	Hypermagnesemia > 2.1 mEq/L	CNS depression, respiratory paralysis; lethargy, coma; bradycardia, hypotension	• Renal insufficiency • Excessive intake from antacids and laxatives, severe dehydration with oliguria
	Hypomagnesemia < 1.4 mEq/L	Tremors, tetany, seizures; positive Chvostek's or Trousseau's signs; tachycardia, hypertension, ventricular arrhythmias; personality changes	• Malnutrition • Alcoholism • Diuretics • Diarrhea • Dehydration

CNS, central nervous system.

Electrolyte Abnormalities: Acid–Base Balance

Electrolyte	Abnormality	Assessment Findings	Causes
Acid–base balance	Metabolic acidosis pH below 7.35 HCO_3 below 22 $PaCO_2$ normal	Tachypnea (Kussmaul's respiration), headache, confusion, drowsiness, cold, clammy skin; vasodilation, which leads to low cardiac output and hypotension	• Renal failure • DKA • Starvation • Poisoning • Diarrhea • Lactic acidosis • Intestinal fistulas
	Metabolic alkalosis pH above 7.45 HCO_3 above 26 $PaCO_2$ normal	Increased neuromuscular irritability, paresthesias; tetany, seizures; dysrhythmias; hypoventilation	• Vomiting • Gastrointestinal suctioning • Diuretic therapy • Cushing's syndrome • Excessive antacid ingestion

DKA, diabetic ketoacidosis.

Factors Affecting Serum Urea: Creatinine Ratio

A. Decreased urea: creatinine (<10:1) *lntha*
   1. Liver disease
   2. Protein restriction
   3. Excessive fluid intake
B. Increased urea: creatinine (>10:1) *P*
   1. Volume depletion
   2. Decreased "effective" blood volume
   3. Catabolic states
   4. Excessive protein intake

Signs and Symptoms of Hypovolemia and Hypervolemia

Parameters	Hypovolemia	Hypervolemia
Skin and subcutaneous tissues	Dry; less elastic	Warm, moist, pitting edema over bony prominences; wrinkled skin from pressure of clothing
Face	Sunken eyes (late symptom)	Periorbital edema
Tongue	Dry, coated (early symptom); fissured (late symptom)	Moist
Saliva	Thick, scanty	Excessive, frothy
Thirst	Present	May not be significant
Temperature	May be elevated	May not be significant
Pulse	Rapid, weak, thready	Rapid
Respirations	Rapid, shallow	Rapid dyspnea, moist rales, cough
Blood pressure	Low, orthostatic hypotension; small pulse pressure	Normal to high
Weight	Loss	Gain

Factors Affecting Water Balance

	Water Excess	Water Deficiency
Intake		
Thirst	Decreased thirst threshold	Increased thirst threshold
	Increased osmolality	Decreased osmolality
	Potassium depletion	Lack of access
	Hypercalcemia	Psychiatric disorders
	Fever	
	Dry mucous membranes Poor oral hygiene Unmisted O_2 administration	
	Hypotension	
	Psychiatric disorders	
Parenteral fluids	Excessive D5W	Deficient replacement
		Osmotic loads Hyperalimentation Hyperglycemia Mannitol Radiographic contrast agents
Output		
Sweating		High ambient temperature
		High altitude
		Fever
Renal excretion	Inappropriate ADH release	Excess excretion
	Appropriate ADH release Congestive failure Decompensated cirrhosis Volume depletion Adrenal insufficiency Renal salt-wasting Hemorrhage Diuretics Burns Hypothyroidism	Central Nephrogenic Potassium depletion Hypercalcemia Lithium administration Declomicin Penthrane

(*continued*)

Factors Affecting Water Balance (continued)

Water Excess	Water Deficiency

Renal disease
  ARF
  Chronic renal failure
  Nephrotic syndrome
  Acute glomerulone-
    phritis
  Nonsteroidal anti-inflam-
    matory agents	

D5W, Dextrose 5% in water; ADH, antidiuretic hormone; ARF, acute renal failure.

Indications for Renal Biopsy

Clinical Condition	Biopsy Indicated	Expected Gain
Orthostatic proteinuria	No	—
Isolated hematuria and/or proteinuria	No*	—
Hematuria and/or proteinuria with ↓ GFR	Yes	D,P,T
Nephrotic syndrome	Yes	D,P,T
Systemic disease with renal abnormalities	Yes†	D,P,T
Classic ARF	No	—
ARF with 1. azotemia >3 wk	Yes	D,P
2. moderate proteinuria	Yes	D,T
3. anuria	Yes	D,T
4. eosinophilia or eosinophiluria	Yes	D,T
Post-transplant ↓ in GFR	Yes	D,P,T

GFR, glomerular filtration rate; D, diagnosis; P, prognosis; T, therapy; ARF, acute renal failure.
* Biopsy may be indicated for insurance, administrative reasons, and so forth.
† Biopsy may or may not be indicated, depending on clinical picture.

Radiologic Study of Kidneys

Diagnostic Test	Purpose
1. Roentgenography	
a. Radiograph of kidney–ureter–bladder (KUB)	a. To detect abnormal calcifications, renal size
b. Tomography	b. To determine renal outlines and abnormalities
c. Intravenous pyelography (IVP)	c. To detect anatomic abnormalities of the kidneys and ureters
d. Retrograde pyelography	d. To assess renal size, to evaluate ureteral obstruction, to localize and diagnose tumors, obstructions
e. Antegrade pyelography	e. To distinguish cysts from hydronephrosis
f. Renal arteriography and venography	f. To evaluate possible renal arterial stenosis, renal mass lesions, renal vein thrombosis, and venous extension of renal cell carcinoma
g. Digital subtraction angiography	g. To visualize major arterial vessels
2. Ultrasonography	a. To delineate renal outlines
	b. To measure longitudinal and transverse dimensions of the kidneys
	c. To evaluate mass lesions
	d. To examine perinephric area
	e. To detect and grade hydronephrosis
3. Radionuclide scintillation imaging (renal scan)	
a. Static imaging	a. To evaluate location, size, and contour of functional renal tissue; may reveal areas of inhomogeneity or filling defects
b. Dynamic imaging	b. To monitor the passage of a radiopharmaceutical agent through the vascular, renal parenchymal, and urinary tract compartments
4. Magnetic resonance imaging	
	a. To determine anatomic abnormalities

General Categories of Acute Renal Failure

Prerenal Failure	Intrarenal Failure	Postrenal Failure
Dehydration	Acute glomerulonephritis	Kidney stones
Sepsis/shock	Severe renal ischemia	Clots
Hypovolemic shock	Chemicals (radio-	Structure malformation
Vena cava obstruction	graphics dyes, commer-	Tumors
Trauma with bleeding	cial chemicals, etc)	Prostatitism
Sequestration (burns, peritonitis)	Certain drugs (ie, anti-inflammatory drugs, an-	Rupture of the bladder
Hypovolemia (ie, diuretics)	tibiotics)	Ureteral obstruction
Cardiovascular failure (ie, myocardial failure, tamponade, vascular pooling, congestive heart failure, dysrhyth-mia)	Neoplasms	Retroperitoneal fibrosis
	Malignant hypertension	Bilateral renal venous occlusion
	Systemic lupus erythematosus	Neurogenic bladder
	Diabetes mellitus	
Hemorrhage	Complications of preg-nancy (ie, eclampsia)	
Gastrointestinal losses (diarrhea, vomiting)	Streptococcal infections	
Extreme acidosis	Vasopressors	
Anaphylaxis/shock	Microangiopathy	
Renal artery stenosis or thrombosis	Hyperviscosity states	
	Hypercalcemia	
	Postrenal transplant	
	Myeloma	
	Interstitial nephritis	
	Transfusion reactions	
	HIV nephropathy	
	Heroin nephropathy	

Common Causes of Acute Renal Failure

Ischemic (prerenal)	Nephrotoxic (intrarenal)
Hemorrhagic hypotension	Antibiotics: aminoglycosides, penicillins, tetracycline, amphotericin
Severe volume depletion	
Surgical aortic cross-clamping	Heavy metals: mercury, lead, *cis*-platinum, uranium, cadmium, bismuth, arsenic
Cardiac and biliary surgery	
Defective cardiac output, including open heart surgery	Hemoglobinuria (from hemolysis)
	Myoglobinuria (rhabdomyolysis)
Septic shock	Radiologic contrast agents
Pregnancy	Drugs: phenytoin, phenylbutazone, cimetidine, cyclosporine
Pancreatitis	
	Organic solvents: carbon tetrachloride
	Fungicides and pesticides
	Uric acid
	Ethylene glycol
	Anesthetics (methoxyflurane)
	Disseminated intravascular coagulation
	Plant and animal substances (mushrooms, snake venom)

Diagnostic Clues in Acute Renal Failure

Urine

- *Urate crystals:* Tumor lysis, especially lymphoma (urate nephropathy)
- *Oxalate crystals:* Ethylene glycol nephrotoxicity, methoxyflurane nephrotoxicity
- *Eosinophils:* Allergic interstitial nephritis, especially methicillin
- *Positive benzidene without RBCs:* Hemoglobinuria or myoglobinuria
- *Pigmented casts:* Hemoglobinuria or myoglobinuria
- *Massive proteinuria:* Acute interstitial nephritis, thiazide diuretics, hemorrhagic fevers (Korean, Scandinavian, etc.)
- *Anuria:* Renal cortical necrosis, bilateral obstruction, hemolytic uremic syndrome, rapidly progressive glomerulonephritis

Plasma

- *Marked hyperkalemia:* Rhabdomyolysis, tissue necrosis, hemolysis
- *Marked hypocalcemia:* Rhabdomyolysis
- *Hypercalcemia:* Hypercalcemic nephropathy
- *Hyperuricemia:* Tumor lysis, rhabdomyolysis, toxin ingestion
- *Marked acidosis:* Ethylene glycol, methyl alcohol
- *Eosinophilia:* Allergic interstitial nephritis

RBCs, red blood cells.

Use of Laboratory Values in Differentiating Acute Tubular Necrosis From Decreased Renal Perfusion

Test	Acute Tubular Necrosis	Reduced Renal Blood Flow
Urine		
Volume	<400 ml/24 hr	<400 ml/24 hr
Sodium	40–10 mEq/L	<5 mEq/L
Specific gravity	1.010	Usually >1.020
Osmolality	250–350 mOsm/L	Usually >400 mOsm/L
Urea	200–300 mg/100 ml	Usually >600 mg/100 ml
Creatinine	<60 mg/100 ml	Usually >150 mg/100 ml
Fe_{Na}	>3.0%	<1.0%
Blood		
BUN:Cr	10:1	Usually >20:1
Responses to Mannitol	None	None or flow increases to >40 ml/hr
Furosemide	None	Flow increases to >40 ml/hr

FE_{Na}, fractional excretion of sodium; BUN:Cr, blood urea nitrogen–creatinine ratio.

Care of the Hemodialysis Access

AV Fistula or Graft
1. No blood pressures or blood drawing from the access limb.
2. Listen for bruit and palpate for thrill each shift.
3. No tight clothing or restraints on the access limb.
4. In the event of postdialysis bleeding from the needle site, apply just enough pressure to stop the flow of blood and hold till bleeding stops. NEVER occlude the vessel.
5. Hypotension can predispose to clotting; therefore, check more frequently for patency.

Dual-Lumen Access Catheter
1. Subclavian and internal jugular vein catheters must have placement verified radiographically before use.
2. A central line dressing is used to cover the insertion site and is cared for according to institutional policy.
3. Both limbs of the catheter usually are filled with concentrated heparin; therefore, *never* inject any other medication into the catheter.
4. *Never unclamp the catheter*—this can cause blood to back up into the lumen and clot.

Comparison of Hemodialysis and Peritoneal Dialysis as Treatment for Acute Renal Failure

	Peritoneal	Hemodialysis
Access	Peritoneal catheter	AV Arteriovenous fistula or graft, Dual-lumen venous catheter
Heparin requirements	Not required	Systemic
Length of treatment	Continuous or intermittent exchanges	3–4 hours, three to five times per week, depending on patient acuity
Complications	Peritonitis, dialysate leaks, exit site or tunnel infections, inability to infuse or drain, hernias	Hypotension, muscle cramps, bleeding, cardiac instability during treatment, clotted accesses, machine malfunction
Advantages	Continuous removal of wastes and fluid, better hemodynamic stability, fewer dietary restrictions	Quick, efficient removal of metabolic wastes and excess fluid; useful for overdoses and poisonings
Disadvantages	Contraindicated after abdominal surgery or in presence of many scars; removal of waste products may be too slow in a very catabolic patient	May require frequent vascular access procedures, places strain on a compromised cardiovascular system, potential blood loss from bleeding or clotted lines

Recommended Antibiotic Dosage in Renal Failure

Antibiotic Group	Method	Adjustment for Renal Failure GFR (ml/min) >50	10–50	<10	Dialysis Supplement
Aminoglycosides Amikacin Gentamicin Kanamicin Netilmicin Streptomycin Tobramicin	I*	12–18	12	24	Yes
Cephalosporins All except Cefoperozone require reduction, but adjustments vary significantly between drugs.					Yes
Cefaclor	D†	100	50–100	33	Yes
Cefadroxil	I	8	12–24	24–48	Yes
Cefamandole	I	6	6–8	8	Yes
Cefazolin	I	8	12	24–48	Yes
Cefoperazone	I	—	None†	—	Yes
Ceforanide	I	12	24–48	48–72	Yes
Cefotaximine	I	6–8	8–12	12–24	Yes
Cefoxitin	I	8	8–12	24–48	Yes
Cefroxadine	D	65–100	15–65	10–15	?
Cefuroxime	I	8–12	24–48	48–72	Yes
Cefsulodin	D	50–100	15–50	10–15	Yes
Ceftizoxime	D	45–100	10–45	5–10	?
Cephalothin	I	6	6	8–12	Yes
Cephalexin	I	6	6–8	12	Yes
Cephapirin	I	6	6–8	12	Yes
Cephradrine	D	100	50	25	Yes
Moxalactam	I	8	12	12–24	Yes
Clindamycin	D	—	None	—	Yes
Erythromycin	D	—	None	—	Yes
Lincomycin	I	6	12	24	Yes
Methenanime mandelate	D	100	Avoid§	Avoid	—
Nalidixic acid	D	100	Avoid	Avoid	—

(continued)

Recommended Antibiotic Dosage in Renal Failure (continued)

Antibiotic Group	Method	GFR (ml/min) >50	GFR (ml/min) 10–50	GFR (ml/min) <10	Dialysis Supplement
Nitrofurantoin	D	100	Avoid	Avoid	—
Penicillins					
Amoxicillin	I	6	6–12	12–16	Yes
Ampicillin	I	6	6–12	12–16	Yes
Azlocillin	I	4–6	6–8	8	Yes
Carbenicillin	I	8–12	12–24	24–48	Yes
Cloxacillin	D	—	None	—	No‖
Cyclacillin	I	6	6–12	12–24	Yes
Dicloxacillin	I	—	None	—	No
Methicillin	I	4	4–8	8–12	No
Mezlocillin	I	4–6	6–8	8	Yes
Nafcillin	D	—	None	—	No
Oxacillin	D	—	None	—	No
Penicillin G	I	6–8	8–12	12–16	Yes
Piperacillin	I	4–6	6–8	8	Yes
Ticarcillin	I	8–12	12–24	24–48	Yes
Sulfonamides and trimethoprim					
Sulfamethoxazole	I	12	18	24	Yes
Sulfisoxazole	I	6	8–12	12–24	Yes
Trimethoprim	I	12	18	24	Yes
Tetracyclines					
Doxycycline	I	12	12–18	18–24	No
Minocycline	D	—	None	—	No
Vancomycin	I	24–72	72–240	240	No

*I refers to alteration in dosage interval in hours.
†D refers to percentage of alteration of usual dose.
‡None means no dosage adjustment is necessary.
§Avoid means drugs toxic in renal failure.
‖No means that hemodialysis does not significantly alter kinetics of the drug.
Modified from Bennett WM, et al: Drug prescribing in renal failure: Dosing guidelines for adults. Am J Kidney Dis 3:155–193, 1983.

Alterations Created by End-Stage Renal Disease Managed by Dialysis and Well-Functioning Transplant

Function	Dialysis	Well-Functioning Transplant
Body fluids	Excess body fluids	Alteration in fluids resolved
	Renal filtration occurs only during dialysis	Acid–base balance maintained
	Metabolic acidosis	
Nutrition	Na, K, protein and fluid restrictions	Possible Na and K restriction for up to 1 yr after transplant
		Possible alterations in diet for hyperglycemia
Hematologic system	Anemia, fatigue	Normal RBC and Hct
	Shortened RBC survival	
	Prolonged clotting time	Normal clotting time
Physical mobility Bone disease	Renal osteodystrophy:	No further bone resorption
	Osteomalacia	Steroid-induced osteoporosis
	Osteoporosis	Possible tertiary hyperparathyroidism
	Osteitis fibrosa cystica	Avascular/aseptic necrosis
	Possible secondary hyperparathyroidism	
Decreased muscle strength	Decreased muscle mass due to dietary limits	Myopathy that improves when steroid dosage decreases and patient's activity increases
	Decreased exercise tolerance	

(continued)

Alterations Created by End-Stage Renal Disease Managed by Dialysis and Well-Functioning Transplant (continued)

Function	Dialysis	Well-Functioning Transplant
Nervous system control	Peripheral, gastrointestinal, and genitourinary neuropathy	Neuropathy will not progress and may improve
	Autonomic nervous system neuropathy	
Hepatic function	Increased risk of hepatitis from extracorporeal circulation in hemodialysis patient	Risk of hepatitis due to azathioprine or cyclosporine therapy
	Increased risk of hepatitis B or non-A, non-B hepatitis from transfusions	Risk of hepatitis B or C from transfusions
		Increased susceptibility to viral hepatitis
Cardiovascular system	Risk of vascular access infection, clotting, exsanguination, and frequent site changes	No need for vascular access
	Accelerated atherosclerosis	Effect on atherosclerotic process uncertain
	Hypertriglyceridemia	Increased cholesterol levels
	Ventricular hypertrophy, heart failure	Ventricular size sometimes returns to normal
	Uremic pericarditis	
	Cardiac tamponade	
Gastrointestinal function	Increased gastric acid production	Increased risk of ulceration
	Increased incidence of diverticulosis	Diverticulosis predisposes to perforation
	Constipation	
Immune response	Increased susceptibility to infection from uremia	Increased susceptibility to infection from immunosuppressive drugs
		Increased incidence of malignancy (especially skin, lymph, and cervix)

Gas exchange	Risk of pulmonary edema, congestive heart failure	Risk of pulmonary infections secondary to immunosuppressive therapy
Self-concept and body image	Dependent on machine and solutions to support life	Dependent on medications to support renal function
	Gradual, subtle physical changes (eg, change in skin color, muscle loss)	Rapid, abrupt early physical changes (eg, cushingoid appearance, hirsutism, gingival hyperplasia, acne)
Sexual function	Impotence	Persistent impotence often secondary to other medicines, (eg, antihypertensives)
	Decreased libido	Libido usually improves
	Amenorrhea	Ovulation and menses usually return (age appropriate)

RBC, red blood cell; Hct, hematocrit.

HEMODYNAMIC MONITORING

Potential for alteration in hemodynamic status as evidenced by change in blood pressure

Baseline BP

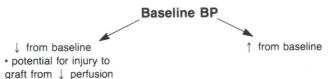

| ↓ from baseline | ↑ from baseline |
| • potential for injury to graft from ↓ perfusion | |

Consider

↓

• hypovolemia
• cardiac tamponade
• response to anesthesia and/or narcotics

Consider

↓

• hypervolemia
• pain
• interruption of antihypertensive therapy in perioperative period

Assessment

↓

• evaluate electrolytes
• CVP
• pulsus paradoxus
• neuro evaluation/level of consciousness
• I & O

Assessment

↓

• evaluate electrolytes
• CVP
• I & O
• degree of pain

Intervention

↓

• treat electrolyte imbalance
• administer vasopressors as indicated
• administer appropriate fluids

Intervention

↓

• treat electrolyte imbalance
• pain control
• administer antihypertensives

FLUID VOLUME STATUS

Potential for alteration in fluid volume status as evidenced by:

Oliguria

↓

Consider:
• hypovolemia
• low output ATN
• obstruction
• dehydration
• ureteral anastamotic leak

Assessment

↓

• check patency of Foley
• compare I&O
• determine baseline
  urinary output from
  native kidneys
• Assess wound for
  urine extravasation
  hematoma
  lymph collection
• evaluate electrolytes
• monitor ECG for signs of
  hyperkalemia

Polyuria

↓

Consider:
• high output ATN with
  potential for hypovolemia
  to develop
• pre or intraoperative over
  hydration

Assessment

↓

• evaluate electrolytes, BUN
  creatinine (especially ↓ K or Na)
• Monitor CVP
• Monitor I&O (with urimeter)

Interventions

• Fluid administration to prevent
  hypovolemia/hypovolemia
• Treatment of electrolyte deviations
• Maintain patency of Foley
• Other interventions dependent upon
  etiology

Immunosuppressive Drugs Used in Renal Transplantation

Drug	Adverse Reactions	Dosage	Comments
Methylprednisolone (Solu-Medrol) (IV) Prednisone (PO)	Increased susceptibility to infection	Initial: 0.5 to 3 mg/kg of body weight, tapered to an adequate oral maintenance dose	Methylprednisolone is given up to 1 wk
	Masks symptoms of infection Peptic ulcer, GI bleeding		An antacid is given while patient is on steroids to reduce the risk of gastric irritation and ulceration; cimetidine may also be used to decrease ulcerogenic tendencies
	Increased appetite, weight gain	During rejection, methylprednisolone may be given in IV boluses up to 1 g/dose	Cardiac arrest can occur if IV bolus of 1 g is given rapidly
	Increased sodium and water retention, which exaggerate hypertension Delayed healing Negative nitrogen balance Adrenal gland suppression Behavior and personality changes		Sodium restriction may be necessary when steroid dosage is high or when fluid retention increases

Diabetogenic effect		
Muscle weakness		
Osteoporosis with long-term therapy		
Skin atrophy, striae		
Easy bruising		
Glaucoma, cataracts		
Hirsutism		
Azathioprine (Imuran) (IV or PO)		Lower doses are given when
Acne		1. Renal function is poor
Avascular/aseptic necrosis		2. WBC is low
Bone marrow suppression: leukopenia, thrombocytopenia, anemia, pancytopenia	Regulated to keep WBC 5,000 to 10,000. Drug usually stopped when WBC is 3,000 or less	3. Given concurrently with allopurinol, which delays metabolism of azathioprine (allopurinol and azathioprine are synergistic)
Rash		
Alopecia	Initial 2–5 mg/kg of body weight	
Liver damage, jaundice		
Increased susceptibility to infection	Maintenance: 2–3 mg/kg of body weight	
During rejection: maximum of 3 mg/kg of body weight, dose not usually increased with rejection		

(continued)

Immunosuppressive Drugs Used in Renal Transplantation *(continued)*

Drug	Adverse Reactions	Dosage	Comments
Cyclosporine (Sandimmune) (IV or PO)	Nephrotoxicity Hepatotoxicity	Initial: 4 mg/kg/day (IV) Maintenance: 5–15 mg/kg/day PO may be used as part of triple therapy regime (prednisone, azathioprine, cyclosporine), or quadruple therapy regime (same as triple therapy plus ALG or OKT3)	Initially, nephrotoxicity and hepatotoxicity seem to be dose-related and respond to dose reduction Long-term nephrotoxicity is a major concern Nephrotoxicity sometimes difficult to differentiate from rejection or ATN Metabolized by cytochrome P-450 enzymes. Drugs that are inducers or inhibitors for P-450 enzymes may increase or decrease cyclosporine concentrations.[6]
	Hypertension Hirsutism Gum hyperplasia Malignancy	Dosage is altered by monitoring drug levels at least during initial period	Trough levels done to monitor and filtrate dosage Administration: liquid form; must be mixed with juice or milk

	Nausea, vomiting, diarrhea Tremors/seizures Diabetogenic effects Anaphylactic reactions have been seen with IV administration		Administer in glass container only, must be precisely measured Risk of anaphylaxis is reduced if slow continuous infusion is given
Monoclonal antibody muromonab-CD3 (Orthoclone OKT3)	Febrile reactions; fever, chills, tremor Respiratory: dyspnea, chest pain, wheezing, pulmonary edema GI: nausea, vomiting, diarrhea	2.5–5 mg/day IV bolus over 30–60 sec, for 10–14 days	Reactions greatest with first dose Reactions occur within 30–60 min To minimize first dose reaction, pretreat with methylprednisolone, acetaminophen, and diphenhydramine hydrochloride Monitor vital signs q15m for 2 hr, then q30m first two doses Have emergency equipment and cooling blanket available
Antilymphocyte globulin (ALG)	Anaphylactic shock due to hypersensitivity to animal serum	Skin test for hypersensitivity to animal serum performed before initial dose	

(continued)

Immunosuppressive Drugs Used in Renal Transplantation (continued)

Drug	Adverse Reactions	Dosage	Comments
Antithymocyte globulin (ATG) Antilymphocyte serum (ALS)	Fever (up to 105°F or 40.6°C) and chills	Dosage may vary	Lymphocytes or platelets decrease sharply with drug administration; therefore, blood work for lymphocyte and platelet counts should be drawn before infusion is started
	Increased susceptibility to infections due to decreased lymphocytes		
Antithymocyte serum (ATS) (usually IV, IM, or deep SC)	IM or deep SC injection site may be swollen, red, and painful, with abscess formation		Usually given only for short period of time to either prevent or treat rejection; not a long-term immunosuppressant
	Difficulty walking if IM or SC injection given in thigh		
Cyclophosphamide (Cytoxan)	Leukopenia, thrombocytopenia	1 to 2 mg/kg (or 1/2 to 2/3 of Imuran dosage)	Given in place of azathioprine when it causes hepatotoxicity
	Increased susceptibility to infections		Administer upon awakening to avoid accumulation of metabolites in bladder while sleeping
	Metabolites are direct irritants to bladder mucosa and may cause hemorrhagic cystitis		Observe for hematuria
			Fluid intake should be encouraged to dilute metabolites
	Alopecia		

| F-K 506 | Infection
Nephrotoxicity
Neurotoxicity
Hypertension
Diabetogenesis | Dosage varies 0.10 mg/kg/day IV
0.30 mg/kg/day PO (given in divided doses) | May be able to discontinue steroids
Monitor renal and liver function
P-450 enzyme system affected |

IV, intravenous; PO, oral; WBC, white blood count; ATN, acute tubular necrosis; IM, intramuscular; SC, subcutaneous.

CHAPTER 6
The Nervous System

Hypothermia

Physiological Reactions During the First 15 to 20 Minutes
of Hypothermia Induction   159
Physiological Effects of the Hypothermic State   159
Normal Temperature Ranges   160

Head Injury

Categories Defining Head Injury Severity Based on
Glasgow Coma Scale Score   160
A Comparison of Upper and Lower Motor Neuron Function   161
A Comparison of Diabetes Insipidus and SIADH   162
Stages of Swallowing Retraining   163
Cognitive Behavior of Brain-Injured Patients and Nursing
Approaches   166
Sensory Stimulation: Planned Nursing Approaches   168

Stroke/Aneurysm

Probable Disabilities Associated with Stroke   169
Common Deficits and Emotional Reactions to Stroke and Related
General Nursing Interventions   170
Comparison of Expressive and Receptive Dysphasia   175
Botterell Classification of Aneurysms   176

Seizures

International Classification of Epileptic Seizures   177
Classification of Status Epilepticus   177
Criteria for Distinguishing Epileptic Seizures From
Pseudoseizures   178
Principles of Treatment of Seizures   179

Spinal Cord Injury

Clinical Manifestations of Spinal Shock   179
Care of a Patient in a Halo Brace   180
Steps in an Intermittent Catheterization Protocol   181
Steps in a Bowel Training Program   182
Skin Care Instructions for the SCI Patient   183
Potential Precipitating Factors of Autonomic Dysreflexia   184
Manifestations of Autonomic Dysreflexia   184
Nursing Treatment Checklist for Autonomic Dysreflexia   185

Responses of Effector Organs to Autonomic Nerve Impulses and Circulating Catecholamines

Effector Organs	Cholinergic Impulses Response	Noradrenergic Impulses Receptor Type	Noradrenergic Impulses Response
Eye			
Radial muscle of iris	—	α	Contraction (mydriasis)
Sphincter muscle of iris	Contraction (miosis)		
Ciliary muscle	Contraction for near vision	β	Relaxation for far vision
Heart			
SA node	Decrease in heart rate; vagal arrest	β_1	Increase in heart rate
Atria	Decrease in contractility and (usually) increase in conduction velocity	β_1	Increase in contractility and conduction velocity
AV node and conduction system	Decrease in conduction velocity; AV block	β_1	Increase in conduction velocity
Ventricles	—	β_1	Increase in contractility and conduction velocity
Arterioles			
Coronary, skeletal muscle, pulmonary, abdominal viscera, renal	Dilation	α	Constriction
		β_2	Dilation

(continued)

Responses of Effector Organs to Autonomic Nerve Impulses and Circulating Catecholamines (continued)

Effector Organs	Cholinergic Impulses Response	Receptor Type	Noradrenergic Impulses Response
Skin and mucosa, cerebral, salivary glands	—	α	Constriction
Systemic Veins	—	α	Constriction
		β_2	Dilation
Lung			
Bronchial muscle	Contraction	β_2	Relaxation
Bronchial glands	Stimulation	?	Inhibition (?)
Stomach			
Motility and tone	Increase	α, β_2	Decrease (usually)
Sphincters	Relaxation (usually)	α	Contraction (usually)
Secretion	Stimulation		Inhibition (?)
Intestine			
Motility and tone	Increase	α, β_2	Decrease
Sphincters	Relaxation (usually)	α	Contraction (usually)
Secretion	Stimulation		Inhibition (?)
Gallbladder and Ducts	Contraction		Relaxation

(*continued*)

Urinary Bladder			
Detrusor	Contraction	β	Relaxation (usually)
Trigone and sphincter	Relaxation	α	Contraction
Ureter			
Motility and tone	Increase (?)	α	Increase (usually)
Uterus	Variable*	α, β₂	Variable*
Male Sex Organs	Erection	α	Ejaculation
Skin			
Pilomotor muscles	—	α	Contraction
Sweat glands	Generalized secretion	α	Slight, localized secretion†
Spleen Capsule	—	α	Contraction
		β₂	Relaxation
Adrenal Medulla	Secretion of epinephrine and nor-epinephrine	—	

Responses of Effector Organs to Autonomic Nerve Impulses and Circulating Catecholamines (continued)

Effector Organs	Cholinergic Impulses Response	Noradrenergic Impulses	
		Receptor Type	Response
Liver	—	α, β₂	Glycogenolysis
Pancreas			
Acini	Secretion	α	Decreased secretion
Islets	Insulin and glucagon secretion	α	Inhibition of insulin and glucagon secretion
		β₂	Insulin and glucagon secretion
Salivary Glands	Profuse, watery secretion	α	Thick, viscous secretion
		β₂	Amylase secretion
Lacrimal Glands	Secretion		—
Nasopharyngeal Glands	Secretion		—
Adipose Tissue	—	β₁	Lipolysis
Juxtaglomerular Cells	—	β(β₁?)	Renin secretion
Pineal Gland	—	β	Melatonin synthesis and secretion

AV, atrioventricular.
* Depends on stage of menstrual cycle, amount of circulating estrogen and progesterone, pregnancy, and other factors.
† On palms of hands and in some other locations ("adrenergic sweating").
(From Ganong WF: Review of Medical Physiology, 11th ed. Los Altos, Lange Medical Publications, 1983)

Format for Mental Status Examination

Attention
Digit span forward and backward
Remembering
Short-term: recall of three items after 5 min
Long-term: recall of mother's maiden name, recall of breakfast menu, events of previous day, etc.
Feeling (affective)
Observe for facial, body expression of mood
Verbal description of affect
Congruence of verbal, body indicators of mood
Language
Content and quantity of spontaneous speech
Naming common objects, parts of objects
Repetition of phrases
Ability to read and explain short passage in newspaper, magazine
Ability to write to dictation, spontaneously
Thinking
Fund of information (example: current president, preceding three)
Knowledge of current events
Orientation to person, place, time (tested as part of arousal, see consciousness)
Calculation: add two numbers, subtract 7 from 100
Problem-solving: What would you do if you found a stamped envelope on the street? What would you do if you smelled smoke in a theater?
Spatial Perception
Copy drawings: square, cross, three-dimensional cube
Draw clock face, map of room
Point out right and left side of self
Demonstrate: putting on a coat, blowing out match, using a toothbrush

(Mitchell PH, Cammermeyer M, et al: Neurological Assessment for Nursing Practice, p 35. Reston, VA, Reston Publishing Co.)

A Method of Grading Responsiveness

Alert: normal

Awake: may sleep more than usual or be somewhat confused on first awakening, but fully oriented when aroused

Lethargic: drowsy but follows simple commands when stimulated

Stuporous: very hard to arouse; inconsistently may follow simple commands or speak single words or short phrases

Semicomatose: movements are purposeful when stimulated; does not follow commands or speak coherently

Comatose: may respond with reflexive posturing when stimulated or may have no response to any stimulus.

A Stimulus-Reaction Level Scale

Level	Description
1	Alert; no delay in response.
2	Drowsy but responsive to gentle stimulation. Confused about either name, place, or time.
3	Very drowsy; responds to strong stimulation with orienting eye movements, obeying commands or localizing, and actively attempting to remove stimulus.
4	Unconscious. Localizes but not successful in removing stimulus.
5	Unconscious. Withdrawal movements to any stimulation.
6	Unconscious. Stereotypical flexion movements to pain.
7	Unconscious. Stereotypical extension movements to pain.
8	Unconscious. No response to pain stimulation.

The Glasgow Coma Scale

Best Eye-Opening Response	Score
Spontaneously	4
To speech	3
To pain	2
No response	1

Best Verbal Response	Score
Oriented	5
Confused conversation	4
Inappropriate words	3
Garbled sounds	2
No response	1

Best Motor Response	Score
Obeys commands	6
Localizes stimuli	5
Withdrawal from stimulus	4
Abnormal flexion (decorticate)	3
Abnormal extension (decerebrate)	2
No response	1

A Grading Scale for Muscle Strength

0 = No muscle contraction
1 = Flicker or trace of contraction
2 = Moves but cannot overcome gravity
3 = Moves against gravity but cannot overcome resistance of examiner's muscles
4 = Moves with some weakness against resistance of examiner's muscles
5 = Normal power and strength

Deep or Muscle Stretch Reflex Grades

4+—Very brisk response; evidence of disease and/or electrolyte imbalance; associated with clonus

3+—A brisk response, possibly indicative of disease

2+—A normal, average response

1+—A response in low-normal range

0 —No response; possibly evidence of disease or electrolyte imbalance

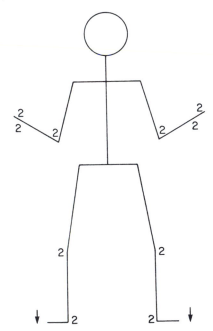

Documentation of selected deep and cutaneous reflexes. Reflexes shown here at major muscle stretch reflex sites are normal and symmetrical.

Testing Superficial and Deep Sensations

Sensation	Stimuli	Dysfunction
Spinothalamic tracts carry impulses for		
Pain	Alternate sharp and dull ends of a pin, asking patient to discriminate between the two (superficial pain). Squeeze nail beds, apply pressure on the orbital rim, rub sternum (deep pain).	• Ipsilateral sensory loss implies a peripheral nerve lesion. • Contralateral sensory loss is seen with lesions of the spinothalamic tract or in the thalamus.
Light touch	Use a wisp of cotton on skin and ask patient to identify when it touches.	• Bilateral sensory loss may indicate a spinal cord lesion. • Paresthesia is an abnormal sensation such as itching or tingling.
Temperature	Use test tubes filled with hot and cold water or use small metal plates of varying temperatures. (Test only if pain and light touch sensations are abnormal.)	• Causalgia is a burning sensation that can be caused by peripheral nerve irritation.
Posterior columns carry impulses for		
Vibration	Apply a vibrating tuning fork on bony prominences and note patient's ability to sense and locate vibrations bilaterally.	• Ipsilateral sensory loss may be due to spinal cord injury or to peripheral neuropathy.
Proprioception	Move the patient's finger or toe up and down and ask patient to identify final resting position.	• Contralateral loss may occur from lesions of the thalamus or of the parietal lobes.

Types of Involuntary Movements

Tremor	Purposeless movement
Resting	Lesion in basal ganglia
Intention	Lesion in cerebellum
Asterixis	Metabolic derangement
Physiologic	Due to fatigue or stress
Fasciculation	Twitching of resting muscles; due to peripheral nerve or spinal cord lesion or to metabolic influences such as cold or anesthetic agents.
Clonus	Repetitive movement; elicited with stretch reflex and implies lesion of the corticospinal tracts.
Myoclonus	Nonrhythmic movement; single jerk-like movements, symmetrical, unknown etiology
Hemiballismus	Flailing movement of extremity; violent movement; not present during sleep; lesion in subthalamic nuclei of basal ganglia
Chorea	Irregular movements; involves limbs and facial muscles; asymmetric movements at rest; involuntary movements may increase when purposeful movement attempted
Athetosis	Slow, writhing movements

A Quick Screening Test for Cranial Nerve Function

	Nerve	Reflex	Procedure
II III	Optic Oculomotor	Pupil constriction (protection of the retina)	Shine a light into each eye and note if the pupil on that side constricts (direct response). Next, shine a light into each eye and note if the opposite pupil constricts (consensual response).
V VII	Trigeminal Facial	Corneal reflex (protection of the cornea)	Approaching the eye from the side and avoiding the eyelashes, touch the cornea with a wisp of cotton. Alternatively, a drop of sterile water or normal saline may be used. A blink response should be present.
IX X	Glossopharyngeal Vagus	Airway protection	Touch the back of the throat with a tongue depressor. A gag or cough response should be present.

Quick Guide to Causes of Pupil Size Changes

Pinpoint pupils
Drugs: opiates
Drops: medications for glaucoma
"Nearly dead": damage in the pons area of the brain stem

Dilated pupils
Fear: panic attack, extreme anxiety
"Fits": seizures
"Fast living": cocaine, crack, phencyclidine (PCP) use

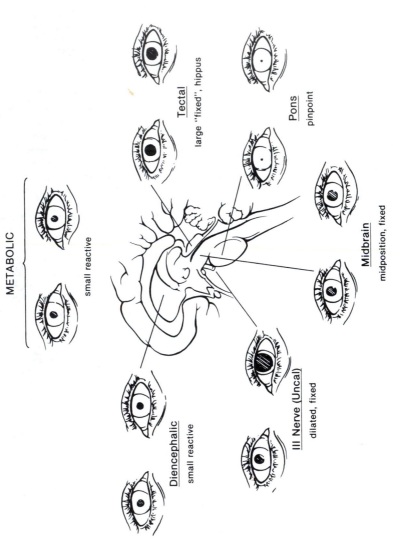

Abnormal pupils. (Adapted from Plum F, Posner J: The Diagnosis of Stupor and Coma, 3rd ed. Philadelphia, FA Davis).

VISUAL FIELD DEFICITS AND NEUROANATOMIC CORRELATES

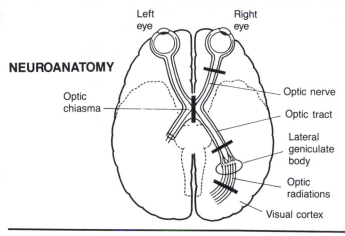

Left
eye

Right
eye

NEUROANATOMY

Optic
chiasma

Optic nerve

Optic tract

Lateral
geniculate
body

Optic
radiations

Visual cortex

FIELD DEFECTS

DESCRIPTION

Anopsia: blindness in one eye;
due to complete lesion of the right
optic nerve, as in trauma.

Bitemporal hemianopsia:
also called central vision; due to lesions around the optic chiasm such
as pituitary tumors or aneurysms of
the anterior communicating artery.

**Left homonymous hemi-
anopsia:** half-vision involving both
eyes with loss of visual field on the
same side of each eye; due to lesion of right temporal or occipital
lobes with damage to the right optic
tract or optic radiations.

Left
eye

Right
eye

Visual field defects associated with lesions of the visual system.

Patterns of Speech Deficits

Type	Deficit Location	Speech Patterns
Fluent dysphasia	Left parietal–temporal lobes (Wernicke's area)	• Fluent speech that lacks coherent content • Impaired understanding of spoken word in spite of normal hearing • May have normal-sounding speech rhythm but no intelligible words • May use invented meaningless words (neologism) or word substitution (paraphasia), or repetition of words (perseveration, echolalia)
Nonfluent dysphasia	Left frontal area (Broca's area)	• Slow speech with poor articulation • Inability to initiate sounds • Comprehension usually intact • Usually associated with impaired writing skills
Global dysphasia	Diffuse involvement of frontal, partietal, and occipital areas	• Nonfluent speech • Inability to understand spoken or written words
Dysarthria	Corticobulbar tracts; cerebellum	• Loss of articulation, phonation • Loss of control of muscles of lips, tongue, palate • Slurred, jerky, or irregular speech but with appropriate content

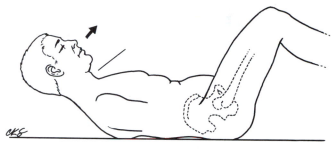

Brudzinksi's sign

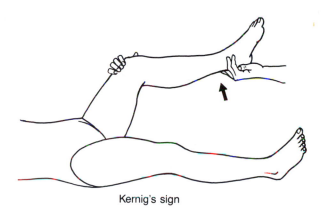

Kernig's sign

Two signs of meningeal irritation.

Neurodiagnostic Tests

Diagnostic Test	What It Is	What It Tells You	Nursing Implications
A. Computed axial tomography, or CT scan (invasive and noninvasive)	A larger scanner takes a series of radiographic images all around the same axial plane. A computer than creates a composite picture of various tissue densities visualized. The images may be enhanced with the use of IV contrast dye.	CT scans give detailed outlines of bone, tissue, and fluid structures of the body. They can indicate shift of structures due to tumors, hematomas, or hydrocephalus. A CT scan is limited in that it gives information only about structure of tissues, not about functional status.	Instruct the patient to lie flat on a table with the machine surrounding, but not touching, the area to be scanned. Patient also must remain as immobile as possible; sedation may be required. The scan may not be of the best quality if the patient moves during the test or if the x-ray beams were deflected by any metal object in or around the patient (ie, traction tongs, ICP monitoring devices).
B. Magnetic resonance imaging (MRI)	A selected area of the patient's body is placed inside a powerful magnetic field. The hydrogen atoms inside the patient are temporarily "excited" and caused to oscillate by a sequence of radiofrequency pulsations. The sensitive scanner measures these minute oscillations, and a computer-enhanced image is created.	An MRI scan creates a graphic image of bone, fluid, and soft tissue structures. It gives a more defined image of anatomic details and may help one diagnose small tumors or early infarction syndromes.	Risk factors for this new technique are not well identified. This test is contraindicated in patients with previous surgeries where hemostatic or aneurysm clips were implanted. The powerful magnetic field can cause such clips to move out of position, placing the patient at risk for bleeding or hemorrhage.

C. Positron Emission Tomography (PET); Single-Photon Emission Computer Tomography (SPECT)

The patient either inhales or receives by injection radioactively tagged substances such as oxygen or glucose. A gamma scanner measures the radioactive uptake of these substances, and a computer produces a composite image, indicating where the radioactive material is located, corresponding to areas of cellular metabolism.

These diagnostic tests are the only ones to measure physiological and biochemical processes in the nervous system. Specific areas can be identified as to functioning and nonfunctioning. Cerebral metabolism and cerebral blood flow can be measured regionally. PET and SPECT scans help diagnose abnormalities (tumors, vascular disease), and also behavioral disturbances such as dementia and schizophrenia that may have a physiological basis.

Inform patient the procedure is very noisy.
Use caution if patient is claustrophobic.

Other contraindications include patients with: cardiac pacemakers, valve prosthesis, bullet fragments, orthopedic pins.

The patient (and any caregivers in the room) must remove all metal objects with magnetic characteristics (eg, scissors, stethoscope).

The patient receives only minimal radiation exposure because the half-life of the radionuclides used is from a few minutes to 2 hr.

Testing may take a few hours.
The patient must remain very still and immobile.

Procedure is very expensive.

(continued)

Neurodiagnostic Tests (continued)

Diagnostic Test	What It Is	What It Tells You	Nursing Implications
D. Cerebral angiography (invasive)	This is a radiographic contrast study in which radiopaque dye is injected by a catheter into the patient's cerebral arterial circulation. The contrast medium is directed into each common carotid artery and each vertebral artery and serial radiographs are then taken.	The contrast dye illuminates the structure of the cerebral circulation. The vessel pathways are examined for patency, narrowing, and occlusion as well as structural abnormalities (aneurysms), vessel displacement (tumors, edema), and alterations in blood flow (tumors, AV malformations)	In preparation for this test, inform the patient as to the location of the catheter insertion (femoral artery is a common site) and that a local anesthetic will be used. Also warm that a warm, flushed feeling will occur when the dye is injected.

After this procedure, assess the puncture site for swelling, redness, and bleeding. Also check the skin color, temperature, and peripheral pulses of the extremity distal to the site for signs of arterial insufficiency due to vasospasm or clotting.

A large amount of contrast medium may be needed during this test, with resulting increased osmotic diuresis and risk of dehydration and renal tubular occlusion. |

E. Digital subtraction angiography (invasive)

In this test, a plain radiograph is taken of the patient's cranium. Then, radioopaque dye is injected into a large vein and serial radiographs are taken. A computer converts the images into digital form and "subtracts" the plain radiograph from the ones with the dye. The result is an enhanced radiographic image of contrast medium in the arterial vessels.

Extracranial circulation (arterial, capillary, and venous) can be examined. Vessel size, patency, narrowing, and degree of stenosis or displacement can be determined.

Other complications include: temporary or permanent neurologic deficit, anaphylaxis, bleeding or hematoma at insertion site, and impaired circulation to the extremity used for injection.

There is less risk to the patient for bleeding or vascular insufficiency because the injection of dye is intravenous rather than intraarterial.

The patient must remain absolutely motionless during the examination (even swallowing will interfere with the results).

F. Myelography (invasive)

A myelogram is a radiographic study in which a contrast substance (either air or dye) is injected into the lumbar subarachnoid space. Fluoroscopy, conventional radiographs, or CT scans are used to visualize selected areas.

The spinal subarachnoid space is examined for partial or complete obstructions due to bone displacements, spinal cord compression, or herniated intervertebral discs.

Instruct the patient as for a lumbar puncture. In addition, advise that a special table will tilt up or down during the procedure.

Postprocedure care is determined by the type of contrast material used.

(continued)

Neurodiagnostic Tests *(continued)*

Diagnostic Test	What It Is	What It Tells You	Nursing Implications
			Oil-based contrast dye: • flat in bed for 24 hr • force fluids • observe for headache, fever, back spasms, nausea and vomiting Water-based contrast dye: • head of bed elevated for 8 hr • keep patient quiet for first few hours • do not administer phenothiazines • observe for headache, fever, back spasms, nausea and vomiting, seizures
G. Electroencephalogram, or EEG (noninvasive)	An EEG is a recording of electrical impulses generated by the brain cortex that are sensed by electrodes on the surface of the scalp.	Analysis of the resulting tracings helps detect and localize abnormal electrical activity occurring in the cerebral cortex. It aids in seizure focus detection, localization of a source of irritation such as a tumor or abscess, and in the diagnosis of metabolic disturbances and sleep disorders.	Reassure the patient that he or she will not feel an electrical shock or pain during this test. The nurse also may need to clarify for the patient that the machine cannot "read minds" or indicate the presence of mental illness.

| **H.** Cortical evoked potentials (noninvasive) | In this test, a specialized device senses central or cortical cerebral electrical activity by skin electrodes in response to peripheral stimulation of specific sensory receptors. The sensory receptors stimulated can be those for vision, hearing, or tactile sensation. The signals are graphically displayed by a computer, and characteristic peaks, and the intervals between them, are measured. | Cortical evoked potentials provide a detailed assessment of neuron transmission along particular pathways. It has value in determining the integrity of visual auditory and tactile pathways in patients with multiple sclerosis and spinal cord injury. This test also may be used in the assessment of a sensory pathway before, during, and after surgery. | The patient's scalp and hair should be free of oil, dirt, creams, and sprays because they can cause electrical interference and thus an inaccurate recording. Inform the EEG technician of electrical devices around the patient that may act as a source of interference during the procedure (eg, cardiac monitor, ventilator). This test may be used in conscious as well as unconscious patients and can be performed at the bedside. The patient must be as motionless as possible during some phases of this test to minimize musculoskeletal interference. Depending on the sensory pathway being tested, the patient may be instructed to watch a series of geometric designs or listen to a series of clicking noises. |

(continued)

Neurodiagnostic Tests (continued)

Diagnostic Test	What It Is	What It Tells You	Nursing Implications
I. Transcranial Doppler sonography (TCD)	This is a test in which high-frequency ultrasonic waves are directed from a probe toward specific cerebral vessels. The ultrasonic energy is aimed through cranial "windows," areas in the skull where the bony table is thin (temporal zygoma) or where there are small gaps in the bone (orbit or foramen magnum). The reflected sound waves are analyzed for shifts in frequency, indicating flow velocity.	The speed or velocity at which blood travels through cerebral vessels is an indicator of the size of the vascular channel and the resistance to blood flow. An approximation of cerebral blood flow may be determined. Cerebral autoregulation can be monitored by observing the response of intracranial vessels to changes in arterial carbon dioxide and to the partial occlusion of the proximal vessels, as may occur in vasospasm.	The test is noninvasive and may be performed at the bedside by the physician or ultrasound technician in 30–60 min. There are no known adverse effects and the procedure may be repeated as often as necessary. The testing is accomplished with the patient initially supine, and later on his or her side, with the head flexed forward.

| J. Lumbar puncture (invasive) | A hollow needle is positioned in the subarachnoid space at L3–4 or L4–5 level, and CSF is sampled. The pressure of the CSF also is measured. Normal pressure varies with age from 45 mm water in full-term newborns to 120 mm water in adults. | The CSF is examined for blood and for alterations in appearance, cell count, protein, and glucose. The opening pressure is roughly equivalent to the ICP for most patients, if done recumbent and no block is present. | This test is contraindicated in patients with suspected increased ICP because a sudden reduction in pressure from below may cause brain structures to herniate, leading to death.

In preparation for this test, position the patient on side with knees and head flexed. Explain to the patient that some pressure may be felt as the needle is inserted and not to move suddenly or cough.

After this procedure, keep the patient flat for 8 to 10 hours to prevent headache. Encourage liberal fluid intake. |

ICP, intracranial pressure; IV intravenous; AV, atrioventricular.

Normal and Abnormal Values for Cerebrospinal Fluid

Characteristic	Normal	Abnormal
Color	Clear, colorless	Cloudy often due to presence of WBC or bacteria
		Xanthochromic due to presence of RBC
WBC	0–5/mm³, all mononuclear	Elevated count accompanies many conditions (tumor, meningitis, subarachnoid hemorrhage, infarct, abscess)
RBC	None	Presence may be due to traumatic tap or subarachnoid hemorrhage (SAH)
Chloride	120–130 mEq/L	Low concentration associated with meningeal infection and tuberculous meningitis
		Elevated level not neurologically significant
Glucose	50–75 mg/100 ml	Decreased level associated with presence of bacteria in CSF
		Elevated level not neurologically significant
Pressure	70–180 mm H₂O	Low pressure associated with inaccurate placement of needle, dehydration, or block along subarachnoid space or at foramen magnum
		Elevated pressure associated with benign intracranial hypertension; cerebral edema; CNS tumor, abscess or cyst; hydrocephalus; muscle tension or abdominal compression; subdural hematoma (SDH)
Protein	14–45 mg/100 ml	Decreased level not neurologically significant
		Increased level associated with demyelinating or degenerative disease, Guillain–Barré syndrome, hemorrhage, infection, spinal block, tumor

WBC, white blood cells; RBC, red blood cells; CSF, cerebrospinal fluid; CNS, central nervous system.

(From Cammermeyer M, Appeldorn C (eds): Core Curriculum for Neuroscience Nursing, 3rd ed, p. Vc7. Chicago, American Association of Neuroscience Nurses, 1990)

Possible Clinical Criteria for Determining Brain Death

Nature of the Comatose State
Must Be Determined

- Drugs must be excluded as a possible cause of the coma.
- The patient may not be hypothermic (ie, body temperature must exceed 33°C, or 91.4°F).
- There must be an appropriate period of observation of patient in comatose state for adequate assessment.

Absence of all Cortical/Brain Stem Function
Must Be Established

- Absence of all cerebral responses to light, noise, motion, and pain.
- Absence of all reflexes or muscle activity unless the reflex activity is determined to be of spinal cord origin.
- Absence of spontaneous respirations with respirator disconnected for at least 3 min, with a PCO_2 of at least 55 mm Hg to stimulate respiratory response. Some institutions do not advocate arterial blood gases and do not recommend complete apnea for 3 min for fear of causing more neuronal death if viable brain function remains. In such institutions, high levels of oxygen are administered passively through endotracheal or tracheostomy tubes for rather prolonged periods without respiration for confirmation of apnea.
- Absence of cranial nerve reflexes: fixed pupils that do not react to light and absence of oculovestibular reflex (caloric ice test response).

In addition, other tests may be required, for example:

- Isoelectric electroencephalogram (EEG). Some institutions require only one isoelectric EEG; others require two, 12 hr apart.
- Absence of intracranial blood flow, as demonstrated by angiography, radioisotope techniques, echo pulsation, or computed tomography scan after administration of contrast medium.

(From Rudy ER: Brain death. Dimensions of Critical Care Nursing 1:183)

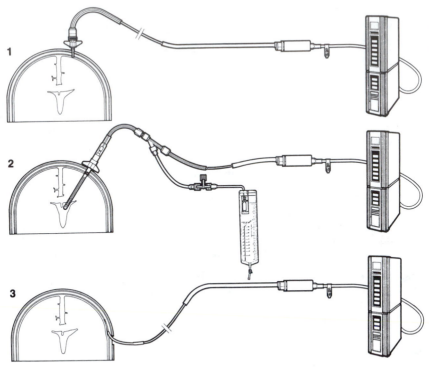

ICP Monitoring Systems. (1) Parenchymal; (2) Ventricular ICP monitoring with ven-triculostomy drainage; (3) Subdural. (Courtesy of Camino Laboratories, San Diego, CA)

ICP Monitoring Risk Factors: Infection

- Duration of ICP monitoring—the most significant risk factor; 85% of infections occur in patients monitored 5 days or longer.
- Maintenance of closed system: intermittent irrigations and tubing–stopcock changes may increase the risk.
- Aseptic technique during insertion and maintenance.
- ICP monitoring technique: intraventricular devices have a higher infection rate.
- Age and diagnosis: older patients and patients with open head trauma or intracerebral–intraventricular hemorrhage.
- Compliance with ICP monitoring protocols.

Modified from Hickman KM, Mayer BL, et al: Intracranial pressure monitoring: Review of risk factors associated with infection. Heart Lung 19:84–91, 1990

Indications for ICP Monitoring

Increased Volume of Brain
Cerebral edema
Trauma
Surgery
Stroke
Tumor

Increased Volume of Blood
Hematomas
AV malformations
Aneurysm
Stroke
Increase in PCO_2

Increased Volume of CSF
Decreased CSF reabsorption
Congenital hydrocephalus

Lesions
Tumors
Abscesses

Extracranial Causes of IICP

- Position of neck, head, and hips
- Cardiovascular instability
- Increased intrathoracic pressure
- Increased abdominal distention
- Decerebrate posturing and agitation
- Metabolic abnormalities
- Nontherapeutic touch and painful procedures
- Extraneous sounds
- Suctioning
- Hygienic measures
- Emotionally charged conversations

Troubleshooting ICP Lines

Problem	Cause	Action
No ICP waveform	Air between the transducer diaphragm and pressure source	Eliminate air bubbles with sterile saline.
	Occlusion of intracranial measurement device with blood or debris	Flush intracranial catheter or screw as directed by physician: 0.25 ml sterile saline is frequently used.
	Transducer connected incorrectly	Check connection and be sure the appropriate connector for amplifier is in use.
	Fiberoptic catheter bent, broken	Replace fiberoptic catheter
	Incorrect gain setting for pressure or patient having plateau waves	Adjust gain setting for higher pressure range.
	Trace turned off	Turn power on to trace.
False high-pressure reading	Transducer too low	Place the venting port of the transducer at the level of the foramen of Monro. For every 2.54 cm (1 in) the transducer is below the pressure source, there is an error of approximately 2 mm Hg.
	Transducer incorrectly balanced	With transducer correctly positioned, rebalance. Transducer should be balanced every 2 to 4 hr and before the initiation of treatment based on a pressure change.
	Monitoring system incorrectly calibrated	Repeat calibration procedures.
	Air in system: air may attenuate or amplify pressure signal	Remove air from monitoring line.

High-pressure reading		
Airway not patent: an increase in intrathoracic pressure may increase PCO_2		Suction patient.
Ventilator setting incorrect		Position. Initiate chest physiotherapy.
PEEP		Check ventilator settings.
		Draw arterial blood gases, because hypoxia and hypercarbia cause increases in ICP.
Posture		Head should be elevated 15° to 30° unless contraindicated by other problems such as fractures.
Head and neck		The head should be positioned to facilitate venous drainage.
Legs		Limit knee flexion.
Decerebrate		Muscle relaxants or paralyzing agents sometimes are indicated.
Excessive muscle activity during decerebrate posturing in patients with upper brain stem injury may increase ICP		
Hyperthermia		Initiate measures to control muscle movement, infection, and pyrexia.
Excessive muscle activity		
Increased susceptibility to infection		
Fluid and electrolyte imbalance secondary to fluid restrictions and diuretics		Draw blood for serum electrolytes, serum osmolality.
		Note pulmonary artery pressure.
		Evaluate input and output with specific gravity.
Blood pressure: vasopressor responses occur in some patients with IICP		Use measures to maintain adequate CPP.
Low BP associated with hypovolemia, shock, and barbiturate coma may increase cerebral ischemia		

(continued)

Troubleshooting ICP Lines (continued)

Problem	Cause	Action
False low-pressure reading	Air bubbles between transducer and CSF	Eliminate air bubbles with sterile saline
	Transducer level too high	Place the venting port of the transducer at the level of the foramen of Monro. For every 2.54 cm (1 in) the transducer is above the level of the pressure source, there will be an error of approximately 2 mm Hg.
	Zero or calibration incorrect	Rezero and calibrate monitoring system.
	Collapse of ventricles around catheter	If ventriculostomy is being used there may be inadequate positive pressure. Check to make sure a positive pressure of 15 to 20 mm Hg exists. Drain CSF slowly.
	Otorrhea or rhinorrhea	These conditions cause a false low-pressure reading secondary to decompression. Document the correlation between drainage and pressure changes.
	Leakage of fluid from connections	Eliminate all fluid leakage.
	Dislodgement of catheter from ventricle into brain	Contact physician regarding appropriate diagnostic studies and intervention. Use soft catheter designed for intraventricular measurement.
	Occlusion of the end of a subarachnoid screw by the necrotic brain	In most cases, remove screw.

ICP, intracranial pressure; PEEP, positive end-expiratory pressure; IICP, increased intracranial pressure; CPP, cerebral perfusion pressure; BP, blood pressure; CSF, cerebrospinal fluid.

Physiological Reactions During the First 15 to 20 Minutes of Hypothermia Induction

Skin: Pallor

Motor activity: Shivering

Pulse: Increased

Blood pressure: Increased

Respiratory rate: Increased

Temperature: May increase initially due to increased cellular activity

Physiological Effects of the Hypothermic State

	Response	Possible Complications
Skin	Decreased circulation leading to crystal formation in cells	Fat necrosis
Vital signs	Diminished	Respiratory acidosis Metabolic acidosis
Urinary output	Increased	
Fluid volume	Hemoconcentration	Embolization
Sensorium	Fades at 34°–33°C	Increased difficulty in determining mental status
Hearing	Fades at 34°–33°C	
Cardiac rhythm	Myocardial irritability below 28°C	Dysrhythmias

Normal Temperature Ranges

Oral	97.6°–99.6°F
	36.5°–37.5°C
Core	98.2°–100.2°F
	36.8°–37.9°C
Rectal	98.6°–100.6°F
	37.0°–38.1°C

Categories Defining Head Injury Severity Based on Glascow Coma Scale (GCS) Score

Severity	Description	Frequency
Minor	GCS 13–15	55%
	May have loss of consciousness or amnesia but for less than 30 minutes.	
	No skull fracture, cerebral contusion, hematoma.	
Moderate	GCS 9–12	24%
	Loss of consciousness and/or amnesia occured for more than 30 minutes but less than 24 hours.	
	May have a skull fracture.	
Severe	GCS 3–8	21%
	Loss of consciousness and/or amnesia occured for more than 24 hours.	
	Also includes those with a cerebral contusion, laceration, or intracranial hematoma.	

A Comparison of Upper and Lower Motor Neuron Function

Neuron	Pathway/Names	Functions	Signs of Dysfunction

Neuron group no. 1, or "upper" motor neurons	From motor area of cerebral cortex to brain stem (corticobulbar tracts) or to spinal cord (corticospinal tracts)	Carries commands for voluntary movement of specific body parts
		
		Carries inhibition commands to control the response of the next neuron pathway
			Loss of voluntary muscle control
			
			Loss of inhibition of lower motor neurons, resulting in:
			  Preservation of reflex arcs
			  Pathologic reflex responses
			  Spastic muscles
			  Increased muscle tone
			  Little or no muscle atrophy

Neuron group no. 2, or "lower" motor neurons	From brain stem or spinal cord to specific muscle groups; names end in the word "nerve" (eg, femoral nerve, radial nerve)	Relays commands from the upper motor neurons to effect voluntary muscle movement
		
		Forms the effector response branch of the reflex arc
			Loss of voluntary muscle movement
			
			No reflex arc activity, resulting in:
			  Flaccid muscles
			  No pathologic reflex responses
			  Decreased muscle tone
			  Significant muscle atrophy

A Comparison of Diabetes Insipidus and the Syndrome of Inappropriate ADH Secretion

	Diabetes Insipidus (DI)	Syndrome of Inappropriate ADH (SIADH)
Clinical manifestations	Increased thirst drive in the awake patient	Lethargy and confusion, leading to coma and seizures
	Polyuria, usually more than 5 L/day	Decreased urine output, usually less than 500 ml/day
	Urine specific gravity 1.001 to 1.005	Urine specific gravity usually greater than 1.025
	Volume depletion, as evidenced by slightly elevated hematocrit and serum sodium levels	Hemodilution, as evidence by decreased hematocrit and hyponatremia
Medical therapy	Appropriate fluid replacement PO or IV or both	Fluid restriction
		Furosemide diuretics
	Supplemental ADH therapy using injectable pitressin or nasal spray solutions of desmopressin (DDAVP)	Drug therapy with demeclocycline hydrochloride (Declomycin), which blocks the effect of ADH on the kidney

ADH, antidiuretic hormone.

Stages of Swallowing Retraining

	Nursing Responsibility	Speech Responsibility	Diet
Stage "0"			
Patient dependent on tube feedings for total fluid and caloric intake	Coordinates tube feedings. Monitors intake and output.	Initiates assessment. Begins oral stimulation techniques.	NPO
Stage I			
Introduction of foods; patient on tube feedings	Coordinates tube feedings in conjunction with treatment sessions by speech therapist (ie, tube feedings after treatment sessions).	Continues oral stimulation techniques. Diet advanced in progressions as tolerated. Instruct nursing personnel in specific treatment techniques for follow through.	Ice chips Slushes Pudding Applesauce Frozen yogurt
Stage II			
Puree with supplemental tube feedings	Monitor and record calorie and fluid intake to determine supplemental feedings.	Supervise one meal daily. Evaluate patient abilities. Apply therapy techniques. Record information on patient status reports.	Puree Soft cooked egg Cooked cereal Puree meat Puree fruit Plain yogurt Puddings; custards

(continued)

Stages of Swallowing Retraining (continued)

	Nursing Responsibility	Speech Responsibility	Diet
Stage III			
Puree food with or without supplemental tube feedings	Monitor calorie and fluid intake. Supervise meals and actually feed patient.	Apply therapy. Instruct nursing personnel in techniques for meal supervision and actual feeding.	Puree, same as stage II
Stage IV			
Soft food; all calories through oral feedings	Supervise 1 to 3 meals daily.	Supervise 1 to 3 meals daily prn. Instruct nursing personnel in therapy techniques. Reevaluate for progression to stage V. Reevaluate ability to swallow thin liquids safely.	Cooked cereals Cottage cheese Ground meat (moist) Cooked vegetables Casseroles Mashed canned fruit Banana Strained cream soup Liquids, if safe

Stage V

Advance to soft or regular diet based on evaluation of test trays	Supervise all meals.	*Chopped* All eggs, cereals, ground meat, bread, potatoes, chopped fruits, creamed pie
	Reevaluate patient abilities for progression of food and fluid consistency.	*Mechanical Soft* Ground meats Soft fruits, vegetables
	Discharge patient from program.	*Regular Diet* No restrictions

Cognitive Behavior of Brain-Injured Patients and Nursing Approaches

Cognitive Behavior Level

1. *No response* to any stimuli
2. *Generalized response:* stimulus response is inconsistent, limited, nonpurposeful with random movements or incomprehensible sounds.
3. *Localized response:* responses to stimuli are specific but inconsistent. Patient may withdraw or push away, may make sounds, follow some simple commands, or respond to certain family members.

4. *Confused–agitated:* response is primarily to internal confusion with increased state of activity; behavior may be bizarre or aggressive; patient may attempt to remove tubes or restraints or crawl out of bed; verbalization is incoherent or inappropriate; patient shows minimal awareness of environment and absent short-term memory.

Nursing Approaches

Levels 1, 2, and 3

A. Assume that patient can understand all that is said. Converse *with* the patient, not *about* him.
B. Do not overwhelm the patient with talking. Leave some moments of silence between verbal stimuli.
C. Manage the environment to provide only one source of stimulation at a time. If talking is taking place, the radio or TV should be off.
D. Encourage the family to provide short, random periods of sensory input that is meaningful to the patient. A favorite TV program, or tape recording or 30 min of music from the patient's favorite radio station will provide more meaningful stimulation than constant radio accompaniment, which becomes as meaningless as the continual bleep of the cardiac monitor.

Level 4

A. Be calm and soothing in manner when handling the patient. Approach with gentle touch to decrease the occurrence of defensive emotional and motor reflexes.
B. Watch for early signs that the patient is becoming agitated (eg, increased movement, vocal loudness, resistance to activity).
C. When the patient becomes upset, do not try to reason with him or "talk him out of it." Talking will be an additional external stimulus that the patient cannot handle.

D. If the patient remains upset, either remove him from the situation or remove the situation from him.

Levels 5 and 6

A. Present the patient with only one task at a time. Allow him to complete it before giving further instructions.

B. Make sure that you have the patient's attention by placing yourself in view and touching the patient before talking.

C. If the patient becomes confused or resistant, stop talking. Wait until he appears relaxed before continuing with instruction or activity.

D. Use gestures, demonstrations, and only the most necessary words in giving instructions.

E. Maintain the same sequence in routine activities and tasks. Describe these routines to the patient and relate them to time of day.

Level 7

A. Supervision is still necessary for continued learning and safety.

B. Reinforce the patient's memory of routines and schedules with clocks, calendars, and a written log of activities.

Level 8

A. The patient should be able to function without supervision.

B. Consideration should be given to job-retraining or return to school.

5. *Confused, inappropriate, nonagitated:* Patient is alert and responds consistently to simple commands; has short attention span and easily distracted memory impaired with confusion of past and present events; can perform previously learned tasks with maximal structure but is unable to learn new information; may wander off with vague intention of "going home."

6. *Confused–appropriate:* Patient shows goal-directed behavior but still requires external direction; is able to understand simple direction; is able to understand simple reasoning; follows simple directions consistently and requires less supervision for previously learned tasks; has improved past memory depth and detail and beginning immediate awareness of self and surroundings.

7. *Automatic–appropriate:* Patient is able to complete daily routines in structured environment; has increased awareness of self and surroundings but lacks insight, judgment, and problem-solving ability.

8. *Purposeful–appropriate:* Patient is alert, oriented, able to recall and integrate past and recent events; responds appropriately to environment; still has decreased ability in abstract reasoning, stress tolerance, and judgment in emergencies or unusual situations.

Reprinted with permission from Hagen C, Malkmus D, Durham P: Levels of cognitive functioning. In Rehabilitation of the Head Injured Adult: Comprehensive Physical Management. Downey, CA, Professional Staff Association of Rancho Los Amigos Hospital, Inc.)

Sensory Stimulation: Planned Nursing Approaches

Sound

- Explain to the patient what you are going to do.
- Play the patient's favorite television or radio program for 10–15 min. Alternatively, play a tape recording of a familiar voice of a friend or family member.
- Another approach is to clap your hands or ring a bell. Do this for 5–10 sec at a time, moving the sound to different locations around the bed.
- During the program, do not converse with others in the room or perform other activities of patient care. The goal is to minimize distractions so the patient may learn to selectively attend to the stimulus.

Sight

- Place a brightly colored object in the patient's view. Present only one object at a time.
- Alternatively, use an object that is familiar, such as a family photo or favorite poster.

Touch

- Stroke the patient's arm or leg with fabrics of various textures. Alternately, the back of a spoon can simulate smooth texture and a towel rough texture.
- Rubbing lotion over the patient's skin will also stimulate this sense. For some, firm pressure may be better tolerated than very light touch.

Smell

- Hold a container of a pleasing fragrance under the patient's nose. Use a familiar scent such as perfume, aftershave, cinnamon, or coffee.
- Present this stimulation for very short periods (1–3 min maximum).
- If a cuffed tracheostomy or endotracheal tube is in place, the patient will not be able to fully appreciate this stimulation.

Adapted from Buss PA, Chippendale JL: Sensory Stimulation: A Guide for the Family of Brain-Injured Patients. San Diego, Sharp Memorial Hospital.

Probable Disabilities Associated With Stroke

Left Hemispheric Stroke

- Right-sided hemiparesis or hemiplegia
- Slow and cautious behavior
- Right visual field defect
- Expressive, receptive, or global dysphasia
- High frustration

Right Hemispheric Stroke

- Left-sided hemiparesis or hemiplegia
- Spatial–perceptual deficits
- Poor judgment
- Distractibility
- Impulsive behavior
- Apparent unawareness of deficits of affected side and therefore susceptibility to falls or other injuries
- Left visual field defect

Common Deficits and Emotional Reactions to Stroke and Related General Nursing Interventions

Common Motor Deficits

1. Hemiparesis or hemiplegia (side of the body opposite the cerebral episode

2. Dysarthria (muscles of speech impaired)

3. Dysphagia (muscles of swallowing impaired)

Nursing Interventions

1. Position the patient in proper body alignment; use a hand roll to keep the hand in a functional position
   - Provide frequent passive range-of-motion exercises.
   - Reposition the patient every 2 hr.

2. Provide for an alternative method of communication.

3. Test the patient's palatal and pharyngeal reflexes before offering nourishment.
   - Elevate and turn the patient's head to the unaffected side.
   - If the patient is able to manage oral intake, place food on the unaffected side of the patient's mouth.

Common Sensory Deficits

1. Visual deficits (common because the visual pathways cut through much of the cerebral hemispheres)
   a. Homonymous hemianopsia (loss of vision in half of the visual field on the same side)

   b. double vision (diplopia)
   c. Decreased visual acuity

2. Absent or diminished response to superficial sensation (touch, pain, pressure, heat, cold)

Nursing Interventions

1. Be aware that variations of visual deficits may exist and compensate for them.
   a. Approach the patient from the unaffected side; remind the patient to turn the head to compensate for visual deficits.
   b. Apply an eye patch to the affected eye.
   c. Provide assistance as necessary.

2. Increase the amount of touch in administering patient care.
   - Protect the involved areas from injury.
   - Protect the involved areas from burns.

3. Absent or diminished response to proprioception (knowledge of position of body parts)

4. Perceptual deficits (disturbance in correctly perceiving and interpreting self and/or environment)

a. Body scheme disturbance (amnesia or denial for paralyzed extremities; unilateral neglect)

b. Disorientation (to time, place, and person)

c. Apraxia (loss of ability to use objects correctly)
d. Agnosia (inability to identify the environment by means of the senses)

e. Defects in localizing objects in space, estimating their size, and judging distance.

f. Impaired memory for recall of spatial location of objects or places

g. Right–left disorientation

- Examine the involved areas for signs of skin irritation and injury.
- Provide the patient with an opportunity to handle various objects of different weight, texture, and size.
- If pain is present, assess its location and type, as well as the duration of the pain.

3. Teach the patient to check the position of body parts visually.

4. Compensate for the patient's perceptual-sensory deficits.

a. Protect the involved area.
   - Accept the patient's self-perception.
   - Position the patient to face the involved area.

b. Control the amount of change in the patient's schedule
   - Reorient the patient as necessary
   - Talk to the patient; tell him about the immediate environment.
   - Provide a calendar, clock, pictures of family, and so forth.

c. Correct misuse of objects and demonstrate proper use.
d. Correct misinformation.

e. Reduce any stimuli that will distract the patient.

f. Place necessary equipment where the patient will see it, rather than telling the patient "It is in the closet" and so forth.

g. Phrase requests carefully, like "Lift this leg." (Point to the leg.)

(continued)

Common Deficits and Emotional Reactions to Stroke and Related General Nursing Interventions (continued)

Language Deficits	Nursing Interventions
1. Expressive aphasia (difficulty in transforming sound into patterns of understandable speech)—can speak using single-word responses	1. Ask the patient to repeat the individual sounds of the alphabet as a start at retraining.
2. Receptive aphasia (impairment of comprehension of the spoken word)—able to speak, but uses words incorrectly and is unaware of these errors	2. Speak clearly and in simple sentences; use gestures as necessary.
3. Global aphasia (combination of expressive and receptive aphasia)—unable to communicate at any level	3. Evaluate what language skills are intact; speak in very simple sentences, ask the patient to repeat individual sounds, and use gestures or any other means to communicate.
4. Alexia (inability to understand the written word)	4. Point to the written names of objects and have the patient repeat the name of the object.
5. Agraphia (inability to express ideas in writing)	5. Have the patient write words and simple sentences.

Intellectual Deficits	Nursing Interventions
1. Loss of memory	1. Provide necessary information as necessary.
2. Short attention span	2. Divide activities into short steps.
3. Increased distractibility	3. Control any excessive environmental distractions.
4. Poor judgment	4. Protect the patient from injury.
5. Inability to transfer learning from one situation to another	5. Repeat instructions as necessary.
6. Inability to calculate, reason, or think abstractly	6. Do not set unrealistic expectations for the patient.

Emotional Deficits

1. Emotional lability (exhibits reactions easily or inappropriately)
2. Loss of self-control and social inhibitions

3. Reduced tolerance to stress
4. Fear, hostility, frustration, anger
5. Confusion and despair
6. Withdrawal, isolation
7. Depression

Nursing Interventions

1. Disregard bursts of emotions; explain to the patient that emotional lability is part of the illness.
2. Protect the patient as necessary so that his or her dignity is preserved.
3. Control the amount of stress experienced by the patient.
4. Be accepting of the patient; be supportive.
5. Clarify any misconceptions; allow the patient to verbalize.
6. Provide stimulation and a safe, comfortable environment.
7. Provide a supportive environment.

Bowel and Bladder Dysfunction

Bladder: Incomplete Upper Motor Neuron Lesion

1. The unilateral lesion from the stroke results in partial sensation and control of the bladder, so that the patient experiences frequency, urgency, and incontinence. (Cognitive deficits affect control.)
2. If the stroke lesion is in the brain stem, there will be bilateral damage, resulting in an upper motor neuron bladder with loss of all control of micturition.

Nursing Interventions

Do not suggest insertion of an indwelling catheter immediately after the stroke.

1. Observe the patient to identify characteristics of the voiding pattern (frequency, amount, forcefulness of stream, constant dribbling, etc.).

2. Maintain an accurate intake and output record.

Nursing note: Incontinence after regaining consciousness is usually attributable to urinary tract infection caused by use of an indwelling urinary catheter.

(continued)

Common Deficits and Emotional Reactions to Stroke and Related General Nursing Interventions (continued)

Bowel and Bladder Dysfunction	Nursing Interventions
	3. Try to allow the patient to stay catheter-free: • Offer the bedpan or urinal frequently. • Take the patient to the commode frequently. • Assess the patient's ability to make his or her need for help with voiding known. If a catheter is necessary, remove it as soon as possible and follow a bladder training program.
3. Possibility of establishing normal bladder function is excellent.	
Bowel	
1. Impairment of bowel function in a stroke patient is attributable to: • Deterioration in the level of consciousness • Dehydration • Immobility	1. Develop a bowel training program: • Give foods known to stimulate defecation (prune juice, roughage). • Initiate a suppository and laxative regimen.
2. Constipation is the most common problem, along with potential impaction.	2. Institute a bowel program. Enemas are avoided in the presence of increased intracranial pressure.

From Hickey JV: The Clinical Practice of Neurological and Neurosurgical Nursing, 3rd ed, pp. 529–530. Philadelphia, JB Lippincott, 1992.

Comparison of Expressive and Receptive Dysphasia

Expressive Dysphasia

Hemiparesis is present because motor cortex is near Broca's area.

Speech is slow, nonfluent; articulation is poor; speaking requires much effort. Total speech is reduced in quantity. Patient may use telegraphic speech, omitting small words.

Patient understands written and verbal speech.

Patient writes dysphasically.

Patient may be able to repeat single words with effort. Phrase repetition is poor.

Object naming is often poor, but it may be better than attempts to use spontaneous speech.

Patient is aware of deficit, often experiencing frustration and depression.

Curses or other ejaculatory speech may be well articulated and automatic. Patient may be able to hum normally.

Receptive Dysphasia

Hemiparesis is mild or absent because lesion is not near motor cortex.

Hemianopsia or quadrantanopsia may be present.

Speech is fluent; articulation and rhythm are normal. Content of speech is impaired; wrong words are used.

Patient does not understand written and verbal speech.

Content of writing is abnormal. Penmanship may be good.

Repetition is poor.

Object naming is poor.

Patient is often unaware of deficit.

Patient may use wrong words and sounds.

Botterell Classification of Aneurysms

Grade	Criteria
Grade I (minimal bleed)	Patient alert, with no focal neurologic signs and no signs of meningeal irritation.
Grade II (mild bleed)	Patient alert with minimal deficits and usually signs of meningeal irritation.
Grade III (moderate bleed)	Patient lethargic, confused, with or without neurologic deficits and signs of meningeal irritation.
Grade IV (moderate to severe bleed)	Patient stuporous or comatose with some purposeful movements. Major neurologic deficits may or may not be evident.
Grade V (severe bleed)	Patient comatose and often decerebrate. Appears moribund.

From Mitchell M: Neuroscience Nursing: A Nursing Diagnosis Approach, p 72. Baltimore, Williams & Wilkins, 1989

International Classification of Epileptic Seizures

I. Partial seizures
   A. Simple partial (consciousness retained)
      1. Motor
      2. Sensory
      3. Autonomic
      4. Psychic
   B. Complex partial (consciousness impaired)
      1. Simple partial, followed by impaired consciousness
      2. Consciousness impaired at onset
   C. Partial seizures with secondary generalization
II. Generalized seizures
   A. Absences
      1. Typical
      2. Atypical
   B. Generalized tonic-clonic
   C. Tonic
   D. Clonic
   E. Myoclonic
   F. Atonic
III. Unclassified seizures

From International League Against Epilepsy: Proposal for revised clinical and electroencephalographic classification of epileptic seizures. Epilepsia 22:489. New York, Raven Press. Reprinted with permission

Classification of Status Epilepticus

I. Convulsive status
   A. Generalized tonic-clonic status
   B. Partial motor status ("epilepsia partialis continua")
II. Nonconvulsive status
   A. Absence status (petit mal status)
   B. Complex partial status (psychomotor status)
   C. Partial sensory status

From Earnest M: Neurologic Emergencies. New York, Churchill-Livingstone (modified from International League Against Epilepsy: Proposal for revised clinical and electroencephalographic classification of epileptic seizures. Epilepsia 22:489. New York, Raven Press. Reprinted with permission).

Criteria for Distinguishing Epileptic Seizures from Pseudoseizures

	Epileptic	Pseudoseizure
Apparent cause	Absent	Emotional disturbance
Warning	Varies, but more commonly unilateral or epigastric aura	Palpitation, malaise, choking, bilateral foot aura
Onset	Commonly sudden	Often gradual
Scream	At onset	During course
Convulsion	Rigidity followed by "jerking"; rarely rigidity alone	Rigidity or "struggling"; throwing limbs and head about
Biting	Tongue	Lips, hands, or more often other people and things
Micturition	Frequent	Never
Defecation	Occasional	Never
Duration	A few minutes	Often half an hour or several hours
Restraint needed	To prevent self-injury	To control violence
Termination	Spontaneous	Spontaneous or artificially induced (water, etc.)

From Konikow N: Hysterical seizures or pseudoseizures. Journal of Neuroscience Nursing 15:22–26.

Principles of Treatment of Seizures

I. Establish the diagnosis and rule out underlying cerebral pathologic condition.
II. Classify seizure type, using clinical and EEG criteria.
III. Select drug of first choice for seizure type.
IV. Increase dose slowly until end point is reached:
   A. Complete seizure control,
   B. Optimum plasma drug level, or
   C. Toxic side effects appear
V. If poor seizure control, gradually withdraw first drug while replacing with second drug of choice for seizure type; monotherapy is preferable to polypharmacy.
VI. If improvement is only partial, other drugs may be necessary.
VII. Adjust dose gradually according to plasma levels, keeping in mind:
   A. Pharamacokinetics of each drug
   B. Potential drug interactions
VIII. If best medical therapy is unsuccessful, refer to specialized epilepsy center for intensive monitoring and possible surgical therapy

From Earnest M: Neurologic Emergencies. New York, Churchill-Livingstone (modified after Meinardi H, Rowan AJ (eds): Advances in Epileptology, p 211. Amsterdam, Swets and Zeitlinger).

Clinical Manifestations of Spinal Shock

- Flaccid paralysis below the level of injury
- Absence of cutaneous and proprioceptive sensation
- Hypotension and bradycardia
- Absence of reflex activity below the level of injury; this may cause urinary retention, bowel paralysis and ileus
- Loss of temperature control; vasodilation and inability to shiver make it difficult for the patient to conserve heat in a cool environment, and the inability to perspire prevents normal cooling in a hot environment
- Reappearance of a reflex that has been depressed after injury is a sign that spinal shock is resolving

Care of a Patient in a Halo Brace

1. Keep wrench taped to front cross-bar so anterior vest can be removed should the need arise to do CPR (some models bend up to give access to the chest).
2. Move patient as a unit. Never use upright bars to move or roll patient.
3. Check skull pins for tightness every day. If loose to finger tightness, report to physician. Pins should not be painful to patient once in place, unless loose.
4. Clean pin sites twice a day as prescribed to prevent infection (usually with Betadine and cotton-tipped applicators).
5. Place rubber cork over tips of halo pins to diminish magnification of sound and for protection of those caring for patient.
6. Avoid placing pillow directly under halo ring. A rolled towel may be used to support the neck.
7. Check edges of vest for comfort and fit by inserting finger between the jacket and the patient's skin. If jacket is too tight, skin breakdown, edema, and possible nerve damage can occur.
8. Check all nuts and bolts for finger tightness daily.
9. Slide pillowcase between vest and patient's skin daily to check for evidence of skin breakdown (serosanguineous drainage).
10. Encourage patient to sleep prone, using pillows under hips and chest and a towel or small pillow to support head.
11. Complaints of difficulty swallowing should be assessed closely. This symptom often indicates an over-hyperextension of the neck and adjustments must be made to the halo immediately to reestablish proper alignment.

A rather new psychological phenomenon has been observed in patients who are having their halo brace removed for the first time, after 12 to 16 weeks. Although patients may have been told repeatedly during the period preceding removal of the brace that their deficits are permanent, many patients seem to attribute the deficits to their halo brace. Perhaps unconsciously, they believe that after the halo is removed, they will improve. When removal of the halo brace does not improve their deficits, they may experience significant depression and begin to grieve for a loss that actually occurred several months earlier. This has been termed *post-halo depression*, and it can be a significant problem. Intervention with psychological support may be necessary at this time.

Steps in an Intermittent Catheterization Protocol

Goal of intermittent catheterization: To eliminate the need for an indwelling urethral or suprapubic catheter, consequently reducing the incidence of urinary tract complications, for example, infections, periurethral abscess, and epididymitis, and to establish and maintain a safe, catheter-free state for patients with neurogenic bladders.

1. Limit fluid intake to 600–800 ml between catheterizations.
2. Catheterize patient every 4 hours initially. When residual urine volumes are consistently less than 400 ml/2 days, decrease catheterizations to every 6 hours.
3. Record voided amounts and residuals on intake and output record.
4. Decrease number of catheterizations as voiding amounts increase or residuals decrease.
5. Catheterize patient every 8 hours when residual urine volumes are consistently less than 300 ml/2 days.
6. Catheterize patient every 12 hours when residual urine volumes are consistently less than 200 ml/2 days.
7. Catheterize patient every 24 hours when residual urine volumes are consistently less than 150 ml/2 days.
8. Catheterize postvoiding every other day for 1 week when residuals are consistently less than 100 ml/2 days.
9. Catheterize postvoiding to measure residual urine volume every third day for 1 week, then once the next week, and then once a month for 3 months. As long as the patient is in the hospital, catheterize postvoiding to measure residual urine volume any time urine infection is demonstrated.
10. Obtain urine culture at start of the program and every 7 days thereafter.
11. When patient begins to void between catheterizations, use an external collector to maintain continence with men. Spiral it around the penis but do not overlap it.
12. Before catheterization procedure, assist patient to empty bladder by Credé or Valsalva maneuvers, anal dilation, or any other method that will trigger voiding for the particular patient. Sometimes tapping or percussing the bladder with one or two fingers will initiate voiding.
13. Notify physician of difficulty with catheterization, increased sediment or mucus in urine, hematuria, or continuous high residuals (over 500 ml).

With permission, from Mitchell M: Neuroscience Nursing: A Nursing Diagnosis Approach, p 202. Baltimore, Williams & Wilkins, 1989.

Steps in a Bowel Training Program

Goal: to attain and maintain bowel continence.

1. Determine bowel habits preinjury if possible.
2. Follow established bowel program. An example of a bowel program is:

   For patients who are being fed (tube feedings or regular food):
   - Colace 100 mg orally or per nasogastric tube three times a day.
   - Dulcolax suppository every night unless the patient has had a bowel movement that day.
   - Milk of magnesia 30 ml orally or per nasogastric tube every other night or even dates unless patient has had a bowel movement that day.

   For patients who are NPO:
   - Dulcolax suppository every other night on even dates.
3. Slush enema may be given every day until peristalsis is present. This consists of giving approximately a liter tap water enema, then holding the container below the level of the bed, allowing the water to return, and repeating the procedure several times.
4. Use bowel program in conjunction with digital stimulation. Digital stimulation consists of inserting a lubricated, gloved index finger into the anal sphincter, using a rotating motion of the finger around the sphincter. The sphincter will slowly dilate as the stimulation occurs. The finger is inserted to about half its length, and the circular rotation is continued for 15–20 minutes until stool passes into the rectum and is then evacuated from the rectum.
5. Once a pattern of evacuation is established, use only digital stimulation if possible, eliminating the suppository. Use only the bowel program on individuals unable to tolerate digital stimulation.
6. Use digital stimulation after each involuntary bowel movement while the bowel pattern is being established.
7. Modify the bowel program according to individual needs as determined by stool consistency.
8. Use Nupercainal ointment or Xylocaine jelly to insert suppository or for digital stimulation if patient is prone to episodes of autonomic dysreflexia. The ointment or jelly may be used in the rectum and around the anal sphincter before insertion of the suppository or finger.
9. Maintain high fluid intake when not contraindicated—for example, in cases of fluid restriction or increased intracranial pressure.
10. Use incontinence pads rather than a bedpan when giving routine bowel care. A bedpan does not work well for these reasons: it is hard and can cause pressure areas over the coccyx; it does not allow access

(*continued*)

Steps in a Bowel Training Program (*continued*)

---

to the anus for digital stimulation; and it can upset the spinal alignment necessary for proper healing in spinal cord-injury patients.
11. Notify physician of prolonged or severe diarrhea, impaction, rectal bleeding, or hemorrhoids.

With permission, from Mitchell M: Neuroscience Nursing: A Nursing Diagnosis Approach, p 201. Baltimore, Williams & Wilkins, 1989.

Skin Care Instructions for the SCI Patient

1. Wear your braces in the car, if you have them, because they will keep your feet where you want them and help maintain balance.
2. When traveling in a van, be sure the wheelchair is secured to the floor and that safety belts are used.
3. Apply elastic stockings or Ace wraps or abdominal binder evenly to prevent skin pressure.
4. Check hands, feet, and legs for swelling. Elevate swollen extremity above the level of the heart. If the swelling does not decrease within 6–8 hours, notify your physician.
5. Use lotion or other lubricating cream if you have dry skin.
6. Protect skin from perspiration, stool, and urine.
7. Wear properly fitting belts, shoes, and socks. Tug at the toes of socks after putting them on to prevent ingrown toenails. Be sure clothing is not tight-fitting.
8. Avoid use of a rubber air ring, because it can cause pressure to the skin and block off the blood supply to the area of skin inside the ring.
9. Avoid nylon underwear, because it retains moisture.
10. Carry coins, billfold, or keys in a place other than a pocket.
11. Items such as a thin metal ashtray should not be rested on your lap, because the heat from the metal may be undetected and cause a burn.
12. Avoid sitting on a vinyl car seat that has been sitting in the sun without covering it with a towel or blanket.
13. Hot water bottles, heating pads, and electric blankets should be avoided.
14. Wear shoes when in a wheelchair to avoid bumping and scraping your feet or toes.

Potential Precipitating Factors of Autonomic Dysreflexia

- Bladder distention or urinary tract infection
- Bladder/kidney stones
- Distended bowel
- Pressure areas or decubiti
- Thrombophlebitis
- Acute abdominal problems such as ulcers, gastritis
- Pulmonary emboli
- Menstruation
- Second stage of labor
- Constrictive clothing
- Heterotopic bone
- Pain
- Sexual activity; ejaculation by a man
- Manipulation/instrumentation of bladder or bowel
- Spasticity
- Exposure to hot or cold stimuli

Manifestations of Autonomic Dysreflexia

- Paroxysmal hypertension
- Pounding headache
- Blurred vision
- Bradycardia
- Profuse sweating above the level of the injury
- Flushing or splotching of the face and neck
- Piloerection
- Nasal congestion
- Nausea
- Pupil dilation

Nursing Treatment Checklist for Autonomic Dysreflexia

1. Elevate head of bed.
2. Apply blood pressure cuff and check blood pressure every 1 to 2 minutes.
   A. If BP is above 180/90, proceed to step 5.
   B. If BP is below 180/90, proceed as follows.
3. Quickly insert bladder catheter or check bladder drainage system in place to detect possible obstruction.
   A. Check to make sure plug or clamp is not in catheter or on tubing.
   B. Check for kinks in catheter or drainage tubing.
   C. Check inlet to leg bag to make sure it is not corroded.
   D. Check to make sure leg bag is not overfull.
   E. If none of these are evident, proceed to step 4.
4. Determine if catheter is plugged by irrigating the bladder slowly with no more than 30 ml of irrigation solution. Use of more solution may increase the massive sympathetic outflow already present. If symptoms have not subsided, proceed to step 5.
5. Change the catheter and empty the bladder.
6. When you are sure the bladder is empty and if BP is:
   A. Above 180/90, call physician immediately.
   B. Below 180/90, proceed as follows:
   Atropine given according to physician's order. If BP rises or fails to subside, call physician immediately. Ismelin, Apresoline, or inhaled amyl nitrate may then be ordered by the physician. Dibenzylene may be used for chronic dysreflexia.
7. Ideally, this procedure requires three people: one to check the BP, one to check the drainage system, and one to notify the physician.

If bladder overdistention does not seem to be the cause of the dysreflexia,

1. Check for bowel impaction. Do not attempt to remove it, if present. Apply Nupercainal ointment or Xylocaine jelly to the rectum and anal area. As the area is anesthetized, the BP should fall. After the BP is again stable, using a generous amount of anesthetizing ointment or jelly, manually remove impaction.
2. Change patient's position. Pressure areas may be the source of dysreflexia.

With permission, from Mitchell M: Neuroscience Nursing: A Nursing Diagnosis Approach, p 199. Baltimore, Williams & Wilkins, 1989.

CHAPTER 7
The Gastrointestinal System

Major Gastrointestinal Secretions Related to Digestion and Absorption

Organ	Cell Type	Substance Secreted	Target of Secretion	Result of Secretion
Tongue	Ebner's glands	Lingual lipase	Ingested triglycerides	Free fatty acids and glycerol
Salivary glands		α Amylase	Ingested carbohydrate (CHO)	CHO changed to simple sugars
		Mucus	Ingested food	Binding of food, lumen protection
Esophagus	Mucosal	Mucus	Ingested food	Lumen protection
Stomach	Parietal	HCl	Pepsinogen, ingested food	Pepsinogen changed to pepsin, other food bonds broken
		Intrinsic factor	Small intestine lumen cells	Vitamin B_{12} absorption
	Chief	Pepsinogen	Ingested proteins	Proteins changed to amino acids
	6 cells (in antrum only)	Gastrin, into bloodstream	Chief and parietal cells	Chief and parietal cells begin and maintain secretion
			Gastric mucosa	Gastric mucosa grows and repairs itself
Pancreas	Exocrine acinar	H_2O	Chyme	Dilution of chyme increases absorption of nutrients
		HCO_3^-	HCl	Neutralization of acid protects intestinal lumen

Organ	Secretion	Acts On	Action
	Enzymes: Trypsinogen Chymotrypsin Elastase Carboxypeptidase	Proteins and connective tissue; other enzymes	Proteins and amino acids further reduced, connective tissue reduced; trypsin converts many other pancreatic enzymes to their active form
	Lipase Colipase Esterase	Fats	Fats changed to free fatty acids and triglycerides
	Phospholipase Nucleases	Cell membranes, DNA and RNA	Cell membranes and nuclear acids changed to lipids, phosphates, amino acids, and small peptides
Gallbladder	Holds and concentrates bile from liver	Ingested fats	Fats emulsified and formed into micelles; with fat-soluble vitamins are now absorbable across intestinal lumen
Duodenum Brunner's glands	H_2O	Chyme	Dilution of chyme increases absorption of nutrients
	HCO_3^-	Acidic chyme	Neutralization of acid protects intestinal lumen
Duodenum and Jejunum Mucosal	Mucus	Chyme	Lumen protection
	Enteropeptidase	Trypsinogen	Trypsinogen converted to trypsin

(continued)

Major Gastrointestinal Secretions Related to Digestion and Absorption (continued)

Organ	Cell Type	Substance Secreted	Target of Secretion	Result of Secretion
		Peptidases	Polypeptides	Gallbladder empties bile into duodenum
			Gallbladder	
		Nucleases	Nucleic acids	Pentoses, purines, pyrimidines, and bases
		Maltase, lactase, and sucrase	Ingested CHO	CHO changed to simple sugars and absorbed
		Secretion, into bloodstream	Pancreas	Pancreas secretes H_2O and HCO_3^- into duodenum
		Cholecystokinin (CCK), into bloodstream	Pancreas	Pancreas secretes enzymes into duodenum
			Gallbladder	Gallbladder empties bile into duodenum
		GIP (glucose-dependent insulinotropic peptide), into bloodstream	Beta cells of the islets of Langerhans	Insulin secretion
			Stomach	Decreased gastric secretions and motility
Colon	Mucosal	Mucus	Feces	Lubrication of fecal material to ease passage
				Lumen protection

Liver Function Tests

Tests	Normal Values	Comments
Protein Studies	**(g/100 ml)**	
Total (Serum)	6.5–8	
Albumin	4–5.5	Albumin is a major part of total blood proteins. It is important in the maintenance of osmotic pressure between blood and tissue.
Globulins	2–3	Globulins are needed for the production of antibodies and to help maintain osmotic pressure.
Fibrinogen	0.2–0.4	Fibrinogen is necessary in the coagulation process.
Electrophoresis	*(percent of 100% total protein)*	Electrophoresis separates the various protein fractions by an electric current. In parenchymal liver cell disease, the amounts of serum proteins is depressed or the ratio of the proteins to each other is altered.
Albumin	53%	
α globulins	14%	
β globulins	12%	
γ globulins	20%	
Prothrombin Time	12–15 seconds	Prothrombin is synthesized to thrombin (in the absence of vitamin K) by the liver. This test is a good index of prognosis, because a prolonged prothrombin time is indicative of severe function loss.
Enzyme Studies		
SGOT	10–40 units	Transaminases are catalysts in the breakdown of amino acids. SGPT is the specific enzyme released by damaged liver cells. LDH is present in large amounts in liver tissue.
SGPT	5–35 units	
LDH	165–300 units	

(continued)

Liver Function Tests (continued)

Tests	Normal Values	Comments
Alkaline phosphatase	2–5 Bodansky units	This enzyme hydrolyzes phosphate esters and is useful in differential diagnosis if jaundice is present. It is excreted through the biliary tract. If it is elevated, nucleotidase and leucine amino peptidase will determine whether elevation is due to biliary obstruction.
Gamma glutamyle transferase	0–30 IU	This endothelia enzyme is found in the liver and closely follows elevations in alkaline phosphatase.
Bilirubin		
Total	0.9–2.2 mg/100 ml (0.8 mg/dl)	This test measures the ability of the liver to conjugate and excrete bilirubin. If the conjugated bilirubin is low and the unconjugated high, a preliver block is indicated. If the conjugated bilirubin is high and the unconjugated normal or low, a postliver block is indicated.
Conjugated (direct)	0.5–1.4 mg/100 ml (0.6 mg/dl)	
Unconjugated (indirect)	0.4–0.8 mg/100 ml (0.2 mg/dl)	
Isotope Liver Scans		Radionuclide scanning of the liver helps define liver cell function and replacement of active liver cells with nonfunctioning tissue, such as scar tissue secondary to cirrhosis, tumors, and abscesses.
CT Liver Scanning		CT scanning is an adjunct that helps define space-occupying lesions within the liver, such as tumors and abscesses. It may be more specific for the finding of tumors and less helpful than the nuclide scanning in the determination of liver cell function.

Common Signs and Symptoms of Type A Hepatitis

Brown urine	Chills
Depression	Headache
Loss of appetite	Right upper quadrant pain
Nausea and vomiting	Irritability
Fever	Clay-colored feces
Weakness	

Indications for Hyperalimentation

Malabsorption

Ulcer disease	Pancreatitis
Chronic diarrhea	Diverticulitis
Chronic vomiting	Alimentary tract fistula
Failure to thrive	Alimentary tract anomalies
Gastrointestinal obstruction	Hepatic failure
Granulomatous enterocolitis	Biliary disease
Ulcerative colitis	Short bowel syndrome
Protein-losing gastroenteropathy	

Inability to Take in Nutrients

Difficulty swallowing	Coma
Neurological weakness	Unable to afford
Malignant disease	NPO 5 or more days
Anorexia nervosa	

Hypermetabolic States

Indolent wounds and decubitus ulcers
Complicated trauma or surgery
Sepsis
Burns

Possible Tests on a Hyperalimentation Panel

Chemistry	Normal Ranges
pH	7.35–7.45
Sodium	135–145 mEq/L
Potassium	3.5–5.3 mEq/L
Chlorides	100–109 mEq/L
Calcium	4.5–5.7 mEq/L
Phosphorus	1.45–2.76 mEq/L
Magnesium	1.4–2.1 mEq/L
Glucose	70–115 mg/dl
BUN	8–22 mg/dl
Creatinine	0.8–1.6 mg/dl
Bicarbonate	22–26 mEq/L
Total protein	5.5–8.0 g/dl

Causes of Gastrointestinal Bleeding

Upper Gastrointestinal Bleeding

Esophageal
  Varices
  Inflammation
  Ulcers
  Tumors
  Mallory-Weiss tears
Gastric
  Ulcers
  Gastritis
  Tumors
  Angiodysplasia
Small intestine
  Peptic ulcers
  Angiodysplasia
  Crohn's disease
  Meckel's diverticulum

Lower Gastrointestinal Bleeding

Malignant tumors
Polyps
Ulcerative colitis
Crohn's disease
Angiodysplasia
Diverticula
Hemorrhoids
Rectal fissures
Massive upper gastrointestinal
  hemorrhage

Diagnostic Findings for Acute GI Bleeding

Complete Blood Count
  Decreased Hemoglobin
  Decreased Hematocrit
  Elevated WBC Count

Electrolyte Panel
  Decreased Serum Potassium
  Elevated Serum Sodium
  Elevated Serum Glucose
  Elevated Lactate (severe bleed)

Hematology Profile
  Prolonged Prothrombin Time
  Prolonged Partial Thromboplastin
  Time

Arterial Blood Gases
  Respiratory Alkalosis
  Hypoxemia

Major Causes of Acute Pancreatitis

Biliary Disease

Gallstones

Common bile duct obstruction

Biliary sludge

Alcohol Abuse

Drugs

Thiazide diuretics

Furosemide

Procainamide

Tetracycline

Sulfonamides

Hypertriglyceridemia

Hypercalcemia

Idiopathic

Postoperative

Ectopic pregnancy

Ovarian cyst

Total parenteral nutrition

Abdominal Trauma

Endoscopic Retrograde Cholangiopancreatography

Infectious Processes

Assessment Parameters in Acute Pancreatitis

History

Alcohol disease
Biliary disease
Nausea and vomiting
Steatorrhea
Urinary discoloration
Hereditary disposition

Clinical Manifestations

Abdominal pain
Abdominal guarding, distention
Paralytic ileus
Fever
Grey Turner's sign
Cullen's sign

Laboratory Findings

Elevated serum and urine amylase
Elevated serum lipase
Elevated WBC count
Hyperglycemia
Elevated bilirubin, SGOT, LDH
(with liver disease)
Elevated alkaline phosphatase (with biliary disease)
Hypertryglyceridemia
Hypocalcemia
Hypoxemia

Diagnostic Studies

Ultrasound
Computer tomography
Magnetic resonance imaging

Ranson Severity Criteria

Evaluate on Admission or on Diagnosis:

Age > 55 years
Leukocyte count > 16,000/μl
Serum Glucose > 200 mg/dl
Serum lactic dehydrogenase > 350 IU/ml
Serum aspartate aminotransferase > 250 IU/dl

During Initial 48 Hours:

Fall in hematocrit > 10%
Blood Urea Nitrogen level rise > 5 mg/dl
Serum Calcium < 8 mg/dl
Base deficit > 4 mEq/L
Estimated fluid sequestration > 6 liters
Arterial Pao$_2$ < 60 torr

Management of Acute Pancreatitis

Fluid Replacement

Colloids

Crystalloids

Blood products

Electrolyte Replacement

Calcium

Magnesium

Potassium

Resting the Pancreas

NG tube to intermittent suction

NPO

Bedrest

Nutritional Support

Pain Management

Non-opiate analgesics

Patient positioning

Major Complications of Acute Pancreatitis

Pulmonary

Atelectasis

Acute Respiratory Distress Syndrome

Cardiovascular

Hypotensive shock

Myocardial depression (MDF)

Renal

Acute renal failure

Hematologic

Disseminated intravascular
coagulation

Metabolic

Hypocalcemia

Metabolic acidosis

Gastrointestinal

Pancreatic pseudocyst

Pancreatic abscess

Gastrointestinal bleed

CHAPTER 8
The Endocrine System

Endocrine System in Summary

Endocrine Gland and Hormone	Principal Site of Action	Principal Results
Hypothalamus		
Corticotropin-releasing factor	Anterior pituitary	Release of adrenocorticotropin
Thyrotropin-releasing factor	Anterior pituitary	Release of thyrotropin
Luteinizing hormone-releasing factor	Anterior pituitary	Release of luteinizing hormone
Follicle-stimulating hormone-releasing factor	Anterior pituitary	Release of follicle-stimulating hormone
Growth hormone-releasing factor	Anterior pituitary	Release of growth hormone
Growth hormone-release inhibiting factor	Anterior pituitary	Inhibition of release of growth hormone
Prolactin-releasing factor	Anterior pituitary	Release of prolactin
Prolactin-release inhibiting hormone	Anterior pituitary	Inhibition of release of prolactin
Pituitary Gland		
Anterior Lobe		
Growth hormone	General	Growth of bones, muscles, and other organs
	Liver	Somatomedin
Thyrotropin	Thyroid	Growth and secretory activity of thyroid gland
Adrenocorticotropin	Adrenal cortex	Growth and secretory activity of adrenal cortex

Hormone	Target	Action
Follicle-stimulating	Ovaries	Development of follicles and secretion of estrogen
	Testes	Development of seminiferous tubules, spermatogenesis
Luteinizing or interstitial cell-stimulating	Ovaries	Ovulation, formation of corpus luteum, secretion of progesterone
	Testes	Secretion of testosterone
Prolactin or lactogenic	Mammary glands	Secretion of milk
Melanocyte-stimulating	Skin	Pigmentation (?)
Posterior Lobe		
Antidiuretic (vasopressin)	Kidney	Reabsorption of water; water balance
Oxytocin	Arterioles	Blood pressure (?)
	Uterus	Contraction
	Breast	Expression of milk
Pineal Gland		
Melatonin	Gonads	Sexual maturation
Thyroid Gland		
Thyroxine and tri-iodothyronine	General	Metabolic rate; growth and development; intermediate metabolism
Thyrocalcitonin	Bone	Inhibits bone resorption; lowers blood level of calcium
Parathyroid Glands		
Parathormone	Bone, kidney, intestine	Promotes bone resorption; increased absorption of calcium; raises blood calcium level

(continued)

Endocrine System in Summary (continued)

Endocrine Gland and Hormone	Principal Site of Action	Principal Results
Adrenal Glands		
Cortex		
Mineralocorticoids (eg, aldosterone)	Kidney	Reabsorption of sodium; elimination of potassium
Glucocorticoids (eg, cortisol)	General	Metabolism of carbohydrate, protein, and fat; response to stress; anti-inflammatory
Sex hormones	General (?)	Preadolescent growth spurt (?)
Medulla		
Epinephrine	Cardiac muscle, smooth muscle, glands	Emergency functions: same as stimulation of sympathetic system
Norepinephrine	Organs innervated by sympathetic system	Chemical transmitter substance; increases peripheral resistance
Islet Cells of Pancreas		
Insulin	General	Lowers blood sugar; utilization and storage of carbohydrate; decreased gluconeogenesis; increased lipogenesis
Somatostatin	Other islet cells	Inhibits secretion of insulin and glucagon
Glucagon	Liver	Raises blood sugar; glucogenolysis and gluconeogenesis
Testes		
Testosterone	General	Development of secondary sex characteristics
	Reproductive organs	Development and maintenance; normal function

Ovaries

Hormone	Target	Action
Estrogens	General	Development of secondary sex characteristics
	Mammary glands	Development of duct system
	Reproductive organs	Maturation and normal cyclic function
Progesterone	Mammary glands	Development of secretory tissue
	Uterus	Preparation for implantation; maintenance of pregnancy
Prostaglandins	General smooth muscle, cell membranes	Contraction–relaxation, enzyme activation

Kidney and Liver

Hormone	Target	Action
Calcitrol	Intestine	Calcium absorption
Erythropoietin	Bone marrow	Erythropoiesis
Renin	Vascular smooth muscle	Vasoconstriction
	Adrenal cortex	Aldosterone secretion

Gastrointestinal Tract

Hormone	Target	Action
Gastrin	Stomach	Production of gastric juice
Enterogastrone	Stomach	Inhibits secretion and motility
Secretin	Liver and pancreas	Production of bile; production of watery pancreatic juice (rich in $NaHCO_3$)
CCK-PZ	Pancreas	Production of pancreatic juice rich in enzymes
	Gallbladder	Contraction and emptying

Cardiac Atria

Hormone	Target	Action
Natriuretic hormone	Kidney	Increased excretion of sodium and water

Adapted from Chaffee EE, Lytle IM: Basic Physiology and Anatomy, 4th ed. Philadelphia: JB Lippincott

Patients at Risk for Development of Endocrine Crisis for Whom the Preexisting Endocrine Disorder is Known

Precipitating factors
    Infection
    Trauma
    Coexistent medical illness (ie, myocardial infarction, pulmonary disease)
    Pregnancy
    Exposure to cold
Medications
    Chronic steroid therapy
    β-blockers
    Narcotics, anesthetics
    Alcohol, tricyclic antidepressants
    Glucocorticoid therapy
    Insulin therapy
    Thiazide diuretics
    Phenytoin
    Chemotherapy agents
    Nonsteroidal anti-inflammatory agents

Adapted from Halloran T: Nursing responsibilities in endocrine emergencies. Critical Care Nursing Quarterly 13:(3):74–81, 1990.

Patients at Risk for Development of Endocrine Crisis for Whom the Preexisting Condition is Unknown

Precipitating factors
    Pituitary tumors
    Radiation therapy of the head and neck
    Autoimmune disease
    Neurosurgical procedures
    Metastatic malignancies (eg, lung, breast)
    Surgery
    Long-term illness
    Shock
    Postpartum
    Trauma

Adapted from Halloran T: Nursing responsibilities in endocrine emergencies. Critical Care Nursing Quarterly 13:(3):74–81, 1990.

Clinical Manifestations of Thyroid Emergencies

Thyroid Storm	Myxedema Coma
Tachycardia	Bradycardia
Hyperthermia	Hypothermia
Tachypnea	Hypoventilation
Hypercalcemia	Hyponatremia
Hyperglycemia	Hypoglycemia
Metabolic acidosis	Respiratory and metabolic acidosis

Cardiovascular collapse due to
  cardiogenic shock
  hypovolemia
  cardiac arrhythmias
	Cardiovascular collapse due to
	  decreased vascular tone

Depressed LOC	Depressed LOC
Emotional lability	Seizures, coma
Psychosis	
Tremors, restlessness	Hyporeflexia

LOC, level of consciousness.
From Halloran T: Nursing responsibilities in endocrine emergencies. Critical Care Nursing Quarterly 13:(3):74–81, 1990.

Clinical Signs and Symptoms of Adrenal Crisis

Aldosterone deficiency
  Hyperkalemia
  Hyponatremia
  Hypovolemia
  Elevated BUN
	Generalized signs and symptoms
	  Anorexia
	  Nausea and vomiting
	  Abdominal cramping
	  Diarrhea

Cortisol deficiency
  Hypoglycemia
  Decreased gastric motility
  Decreased vascular tone
  Hypercalcemia
	Tachycardia
	  Orthostatic hypotension
	  Headache, lethargy
	  Fatigue, weakness
	  Hyperkalemic ECG changes
	  Hyperpigmentation

BUN, blood urea nitrogen; ECG, electrocardiograph.
Adapted from Halloran T: Nursing responsibilities in endocrine emergencies. Critical Care Nursing Quarterly 13:(3):74–81, 1990.

Comparison of Usual Clinical Manifestations of Hyperosmolar Hyperglycemic Nonketotic Coma and Diabetic Ketoacidosis

Hyperosmolar Coma	Diabetic Ketoacidosis

Hyperosmolar Coma

1. Patient has Type II diabetes and may be treated by diet alone, diet and an oral hypoglycemic agent, or diet and insulin therapy
2. Patient usually more than 40 years of age
3. Insidious onset
4. Symptoms include
   a. Slight drowsiness, insidious stupor or frequent coma
   b. Polyuria for 2 days to 2 weeks before clinical presentation
   c. Absence of hyperventilation, no breath odor
   d. Extreme volume depletion (dehydration, hypovolemia)
   e. Serum glucose 600 mg/dl to 2400 mg/dl
   f. Occasional gastrointestinal symptoms
   g. Hypernatremia
   h. Failure of thirst mechanism leading to inadequate water ingestion
   i. High serum osmolarity with minimal CNS symptoms (disorientation, focal seizures)
   j. Impaired renal function
   k. HCO_3 level greater than 16 mEq/L
   l. CO_2 level normal
   m. Anion gap less than 7 mEq/L
   n. Usually normal serum potassium
   o. Ketonemia absent
   p. Lack of acidosis
   q. High mortality rate

Diabetic Ketoacidosis

1. Patient has type I, insulin-dependent diabetes
2. Patient usually less than 40 years of age
3. Usually rapid onset
4. Symptoms include
   a. Drowsiness, stupor, coma
   b. Polyuria for 1 to 3 days prior to clinical presentation
   c. Hyperventilation with possible Kussmaul breathing pattern, "fruity" breath odor
   d. Extreme volume depletion (dehydration, hypovolemia)
   e. Serum glucose 300 mg/dl to 1000 mg/dl
   f. Abdominal pain, nausea, vomiting, and diarrhea
   g. Mild hyponatremia
   h. Polydipsia for 1 to 3 days
   i. High serum osmolarity
   j. Impaired renal function
   k. HCO_3 level less than 10 mEq/L
   l. CO_2 level less than 10 mEq/L
   m. Anion gap greater than 7 mEq/L
   n. Extreme hypokalemia
   o. Ketonemia present
   p. Moderate to severe acidosis
   q. High recovery rate

CHAPTER 9
Multisystem Conditions

Acquired Immunodeficiency Syndrome

Recovery from Anesthesia

Risk Factors for Septic Shock

Host Factors	Treatment-Related Factors
Extremes of age	Use of invasive catheters
Malnutrition	Surgical procedures
General debilitation	Traumatic or thermal wounds
Chronic illness	Invasive diagnostic procedures
Drug or alcohol abuse	Drugs (antibiotics, cytotoxic agents, steroids)
Neutropenia	
Spleenectomy	
Multiple organ failure	

Clinical Manifestations of Septic Shock

Hyperdynamic Shock	Hypodynamic Shock
Hypotension	Hypotension
Tachycardia	Tachycardia
Tachypnea	Tachypnea
Respiratory alkalosis	Metabolic acidosis
High cardiac output with low SVR	Low CO with high SVR
Warm, flushed skin	Cool, pale skin
Hyperthermia/hypothermia	Hypothermia
Altered mental status	Worsening mental status
Polyuria	Other organ and cellular dysfunction (eg, oliguria, DIC, ARDS)
Increased WBCs	
Hyperglycemia	Decreased WBCs
	Hypoglycemia

SVR, systemic vascular resistance; WBCs, white blood cells; CO, cardiac output; DIC, disseminated intravascular coagulation; ARDS, adult respiratory distress syndrome.

Physiologic Data Helpful in Diagnosing Sepsis

1. Cultures: from blood, sputum, urine, surgical or nonsurgical wounds, sinuses, and invasive lines. Positive results are not necessary for diagnosis

2. CBC: WBCs usually will be elevated, may decrease with progression of shock

3. SMA-7: hyperglycemia may be evident, followed by hypoglycemia in later stages

4. Arterial blood gases: respiratory alkalosis present in sepsis (pH >7.45, pCO_2 <35), with mild hypoxemia (PO_2 <80)

5. CT Scan: may be needed to identify sites of potential abscesses

6. Chest and abdominal radiographs: may reveal infectious processes

Equipment-Related Sources for Infection

Intravascular catheters	Intracranial bolts, catheters
Endotracheal/tracheostomy tubes	Orthopedic hardware
Indwelling urinary catheters	Nasogastric tubes
Surgical wound drains	Gastrointestinal tubes

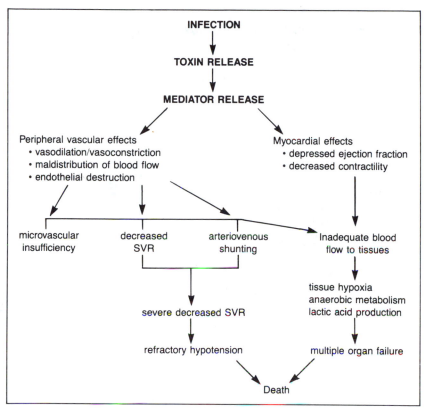

Pathophysiologic cardiovascular events which occur in the presence of septic shock.

Complications of Septic Shock

Adult respiratory distress syndrome
Disseminated intravascular coagulation
Multiple organ failure

Management Highlights for Septic Shock

Definitive therapies
Identify and eliminate the source of infection
Multiple broad-spectrum antibiotics
Supportive therapies
Restore intravascular volume
Maintain adequate cardiac output
Ensure adequate ventilation and oxygenation
Provide appropriate metabolic environment
Investigational therapies
Antihistamines
Monoclonal antibodies to:
Endotoxin and exotoxin
Tumor necrosis factor
Complement factors
Naloxone
Neutrophil inhibitors
Prostaglandin inhibitors (nonsteroidal anti-inflammatory drugs)
Steroids

Laboratory Findings in Acute Disseminated Intravascular Coagulation (DIC)

Test	Normal Value	Value in DIC
Prothrombin time	11–15 seconds	Prolonged
Partial thromboplastin time	39–48 seconds	Prolonged
Thrombin time	10–13 seconds	Usually prolonged
Fibrinogen level	200–400 mg/100 ml	Decreased
Antithrombin III levels	89%–120%	Decreased
Platelet count	150,000–400,000/mm^3	Decreased
Fibrin degradation products	<10	Increased
Plasminogen levels		Decreased

Characteristics of Burns of Various Depths

Depth	Tissues Involved	Usual Cause	Characteristics	Pain	Healing
Superficial partial-thickness (first degree)	Minimal epithelial damage	Sun	Dry No blisters Pinkish red Blanches with pressure	Painful	About 5 days
Superficial partial-thickness (second degree)	Epidermis, minimal dermis	Flash Hot liquids	Moist Pinkish or mottled red Blisters Some blanching	Pain Hyperesthetic	About 21 days, minimal scarring
Deep dermal partial-thickness (second degree)	Entire epidermis, part of dermis, epidermal-lined hair and sweat glands intact	Above plus hot solids, flame, and intense radiant injury	Dry, pale, waxy No blanching	Sensitive to pressure	Prolonged; late hypertrophic scarring; marked contracture formation
Full-thickness (third degree)	All of above, and portion of subcutaneous fat; may involve connective tissue, muscle, bone	Sustained flame, electrical, chemical, and steam	Leathery, cracked avascular, pale yellow to brown to charred	Little pain	Cannot self-regenerate; needs grafting

From Burgess C: Initial management of a patient with extensive burn injury. *Critical Care Nursing Clinics of North America* 3(2):167, 1991.

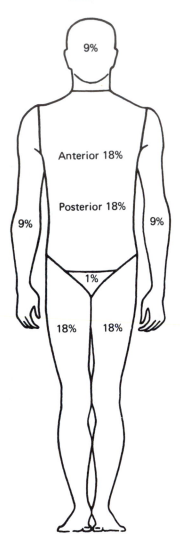

The "rule of nines" method for determining percentage of body area with burn injury.

Formulas for Fluid Replacement/Resuscitation

	First 24 Hours			Second 24 Hours		
	Electrolyte	*Colloid*	*Glucose in Water*	*Electrolyte*	*Colloid*	*Glucose in Water*
Burn budget of F.D. Moore	1,000–4,000 ml lactated Ringer's and 1,200 ml 0.5N saline	7.5% of body weight	1,500–5,000 ml	1,000–4,000 ml lactated Ringer's and 1200 ml 0.5N saline	2.5% of body weight	1,500–5,000 ml
Evans	Normal saline, 1 ml/kg/% burn	1.0 ml/kg/% burn	2,000 ml	One-half of first–24-hr requirement	One-half of first-hour requirement	2,000 ml
Brooke	Lactated Ringer's, 1.5 ml/kg/% burn	0.5 ml/kg/% burn	2,000 ml	One-half to three-quarters of first–24-hr requirement	One-half of three-quarters of first–24-hr requirement	2,000 ml
Parkland	Lactated Ringer's 4 ml/kg/% burn				20%–60% of calculated plasma volume	
Hypertonic sodium solution	Volume to maintain urine output at 30 ml/hr (fluid contains 250 mEq Na/liter)			One-third of salt solution orally, up to 3,500 ml limit		

(*continued*)

Formulas for Fluid Replacement/Resuscitation (continued)

	First 24 Hours			Second 24 Hours		
	Electrolyte	Colloid	Glucose in Water	Electrolyte	Colloid	Glucose in Water
Modified Brooke	Lactated Ringer's 2 ml/kg/% burn				0.3–0.5 ml/kg/% burn	Goal: maintain adequate urinary output
Burnett Burn Center	Isotonic or hypertonic alkaline sodium solution/% burn/kg			$n_{5/4}$ NS maintenance	Colloid 0.5 ml/% burn/kg	D_5W (% burn) (TBSAm^2)

Topical Antimicrobial Agents for Burn Wound Management

Agent	Indications	Nursing Considerations
Mafenide acetate (Sulfamylon)	Active agent against most gram-positive and gram-negative wound pathogens; drug of choice for electrical and ear burns	Apply once or twice daily with sterile glove; do not use dressings that reduce effectiveness and cause maceration; monitor respiratory rate, electrolyte values, and arterial pH for evidence of metabolic acidosis; painful on application to partial-thickness burns for about 30 min
Silver nitrate	Effective against wide spectrum of common wound pathogens and candidal infections; used in patients with sulfa allergy or toxic epidermal necrolysis. Poor penetration of eschar	Apply 0.5% solution wet dressings twice or three times a day; ensure that dressings remain moist by wetting every 2 hours; preserve solution in a light-resistant container; protect walls, floors, etc., with plastic to prevent staining; monitor for hyponatremia and hypochloremia
Silver sulfadiazine	Active against a wide spectrum of microbial pathogens; use with caution in patients with impaired renal or hepatic function	Apply once or twice daily with a sterile gloved hand; leave wounds exposed or wrap lightly with gauze dressings; painless

From Duncan DJ, Driscoll DM: Burn wound management. Critical Care Nursing Clinics of North America 3(2):205, 1991.

Toxic Syndromes

Syndrome	Symptoms	Common Causes
Cholinergic	Decreased vital signs, excessive salivation, lacrimation, urination, emesis and diaphoresis, central nervous system depression, muscle fasiculations, pulmonary edema, miosis, bradycardia, and seizures	Organophosphate and carbamate insecticides, physostigmine, some mushrooms
Opiate/sedative hypnotic	Decreased vital signs, coma, respiratory depression, miosis, hypotension, bradycardia, decreased bowel sounds, pulmonary edema (propoxyphene may cause seizures)	Narcotics, benzodiazepines, barbiturates, ethanol, clonidine, methaqualone
Anticholinergic	Delirium, dry, flushed skin, dilated pupils, elevated temperature, urinary retention, decreased bowel sounds, tachycardia, seizures	Antihistamines, atropine, antidepressant agents, some plants and mushrooms
Sympathomimetic	Delusions, paranoia, tachycardia, hypertension, mydriasis, seizures	Cocaine, theophyllin, caffeine, LSD, amphetamines, phenypropanolamine
Withdrawal	Diarrhea, mydriasis, tachycardia, hallucinations, cramps	Alcohol, barbiturates, narcotics, benzodiazepines

Charcoal-Adsorbed Drugs and Substances

Acetaminophen	Pentobarbital
Amitriptyline	Phenol
Amphetamines	Propoxyphene
Codeine	Salicylates
Morphine	Strychnine
N-acetylcysteine	Theophylline

Substances Not Well Adsorbed by Charcoal

Acids	Ferrous sulfate
Alkalis	Lithium
Ethanol	Potassium chloride

Antidotes

Toxin	Antidote
Opiates	Naloxone
Methanol, ethylene glycol	Ethanol
Anticholinergics	Physostigmine
Organophosphates or carbamate insecticides	Atropine
	Pyridoxine
β-Blockers	Glucagon
Digitalis, glycosides	Digoxin-specific antibody fragments
Benzodiazepines	Flumazenil
Carbon monoxide	Oxygen
Nitrites	Methylene blue
Acetaminophen	N-acetylcysteine (Mucomyst)
Cyanide	Amyl nitrite
	Sodium nitrite
	Sodium thiosulfate
Calcium channel blockers	Calcium gluconate

Commonly Observed Poisonings

Substance/Examples	Nursing Assessment	Diagnostic	Intervention	Comments
Benzodiazepines Diazepam (Valium) Chlordiazepoxide (Librium) Flurazepam (Dalmane) Clorazepate (Tranxene) Oxazepam (Serax)	Vital signs: hypotension, tachycardia, respiratory depression Neurologic: ataxia, lethargy, slurred speech	Plasma levels not usually clinically useful	Supportive care: 1. airway 2. breathing 3. circulation Prevention of absorption: 1. lavage 2. activated charcoal 3. cathartic Fluids for hypotension Antidotes: Flumazenil has reversed coma and respiratory depression in severely poisoned patients, contraindicated in tricyclic antidepressant overdose	Benzodiazepines cause CNS depression effects. Because of their long half-life, these drugs may cause prolonged drowsiness in the overdose situation. Fatalities are unlikely from the ingestion of these agents alone, but frequently they are involved in the multiple overdose, most notably with alcohol. Ingestions of 500–1,500 mg have occurred with only minor toxicity. Physical dependence can occur with chronic ingestion; therefore, withdrawal may be anticipated if a person arrives with an acute oral benzodiazepine overdose.

Propoxyphene

Darvon
Darvon compound
Darvocet N-100

Vital signs: hypotension, respiratory depression
CV:
cardiac dysrhythmias

Neurologic:
CNS depression, drowsiness progressing to coma, convulsions, pinpoint pupils

Arterial blood gases
Propoxyphene levels are not clinically useful

Supportive care:
1. airway
2. breathing
3. circulation

Prevention of absorption:
1. lavage
2. activated charcoal
3. cathartic

Cardiac monitoring

Seizure precaution

Antidote: naloxone

Propoxyphene is a synthetic narcotic found in a variety of preparations, and acts directly on the CNS. Its rapid action allows for observable symptoms within 30 min of ingestion, and effects may be exhibited for 8–12 hr. A diagnostic clue to propoxyphene overdose is that the person will present with seizures and pinpoint pupils. The propensity toward seizures makes lavage preferable to ipecac. Large amounts of naloxone have been required for reversal of the effects of propoxyphene overdose. Most deaths occur within first 2 hr of ingestion, many within 15 min.

(continued)

Commonly Observed Poisonings (continued)

Substance/Examples	Nursing Assessment	Diagnostic	Intervention	Comments
Iron				
Multivitamin with iron	Iron toxicity is best described in four distinct phases:	Serum iron total iron binding capacity	Supportive care:	Iron is found in a number of preparations, including multivitamins with iron and prenatal vitamins. Iron has a direct effect on the gastrointestinal mucosa. In less than 2 hr, there can be severe hemorrhagic necrosis with large losses of blood and fluid. The plasma iron concentration and total iron-binding capacity may vary and are regulated by hemoglobin synthesis. Careful calculations must be made as to the amount of elemental iron ingested.
Ferrous gluconate		Abdominal radiograph	1. airway	
Intron	1. Phase I (30 min– 2 hr)	Electrolytes	2. breathing	
Fergon		White blood cell count	3. circulation (check for hypovolemia)	
Ferrous sulfate	GI:	Blood glucose		
Mol-iron	hemorrhagic gastritis, vomiting, diarrhea	Type and cross-matching for blood	Prevention of absorption:	
Feosol			1. ipecac/lavage	
Fer-In-Sol	CNS:		2. charcoal	
Ferous fumarate	lethargy, coma		3. cathartic (unless pt already has diarrhea)	
	2. Phase II (up to 12 hr after exposure)		Antidotes/chelation	
	Deceptive period of improvement and stabilization; stage may be brief		Deferoxamine Indications:	
	3. Phase III (12–48 hr)		1. Peak serum iron levels above 350 µg/dl	
	GI:		2. symptomatic patients	
	hematemesis, melena, GI perforation		a. hypotension	
			b. bleeding	
	CNS:		c. protracted vomiting	
	lethargy, coma, seizures		Replace fluid loss aggressively	

CV:
vascular collapse, cyanosis, pulmonary edema
Metabolic:
acidosis, hypoglycemia
Liver/kidney: coagulation defects, hepatorenal failure
4. Phase 4 (2–4 days) possible hepatic necrosis

Amphetamines:

Diet pills
Illicit drugs (MDA, MMDA, "Ice")
Methyl phenidate (Cylert)

Vital signs: hypothermia, hyperventilation, hypertension, tachycardia
CV: myocardial stimulation, dysrhythmias
Neurologic: hyperactivity, restlessness, seizures
GI: nausea, vomiting, diarrhea, anorexia

Urine drug screen for amphetamine

Supportive care:
1. airway
2. breathing
3. circulation
Prevention of absorption:
1. lavage
2. activated charcoal
3. cathartic
Cardiac monitoring
Seizure precautions
Nitroprusside for severe hypertension

Used to treat narcolepsy and attention deficit disorder and hyperkinetic syndrome in children, amphetamines also play a role as street drugs. "Ice" is a new form of methamphetamine that is gaining popularity in Hawaii and the West Coast of the United States.

(continued)

Commonly Observed Poisonings (continued)

Substance/Examples	Nursing Assessment	Diagnostic	Intervention	Comments
Amphetamines (continued):				
	Fluid–electrolyte: hypokalemia, hyperkalemia, dehydration Psychiatric: aggressive behavior, delusions		External cooling for hyperthermia Calm environment	

Hydrocarbons	Vital signs: respiratory distress cyanosis, tachypnea
	
	Neurologic: the volatile aromatic hydrocarbons induce higher degrees of CNS toxicity, and their effects may include lethargy, irritability, dizziness, stupor, and coma
	
	GI: irritations of the mouth, burning sensation in the mucous membranes of mouth and esophagus, nausea and vomiting
		Baseline chest radiograph
		
		Arterial blood gases
			Supportive care:
			1. airway
			2. breathing
			3. circulation
			
			Prevention of absorption:
			1. ipecac is recommended in the alert patient with ingestion of:
			  a. large amounts of petroleum distillates
			  b. petroleum distillates with seriously toxic additives (heavy metals, insecticides)
				The most serious toxic effect after ingestion is aspiration pneumonitis. Ingestion of low-viscosity hydrocarbons poses the greatest risk of aspiration and toxicity. Intentional inhalation may result in cardiac dysrhythmias, respiratory arrest, and CNS toxicity. Gastric emptying is not indicated unless there is a history of large ingestion (intentional poisoning) or ingestion of hydrocarbons that may produce renal, liver

CV:
dysrhythmia
Dermal:
skin irritation
Ocular:
corneal burns

c. halogenated aromatic hydrocarbons
d. do not induce emesis for mineral seal oil, signal oil, or furniture polish
2. lavage in patients who require decontamination but are too obtunded to take ipecac
3. charcoal
4. saline cathartics

Cardiac monitor in symptomatic patients

Positive end-expiratory pressure may be necessary to maintain adequate oxygenation

Decontamination eye exposure: irrigate 15 min with tepid water

Dermal-wash area with soap and water

Steroids are not useful

Antibiotics are to be used only if indicated

CNS, or pulmonary toxicity (halogenated hydrocarbons or petroleum distillates with additives).

(*continued*)

Commonly Observed Poisonings *(continued)*

Substance/Examples	Nursing Assessment	Diagnostic	Intervention	Comments
LSD Morning glory seeds	HEENT: mydriasis and impaired color preception CV: hypertension, hypotension, tachycardia Neurologic: acute anxiety, hallucination, fluctuations in mood, paranoia, psychotic reactions, flashbacks GI: vomiting diarrhea Temperature regulation: hyperthermia	Urine drug screen	Supportive care 1. airway 2. breathing 3. circulation Prevention of absorption: 1. activated charcoal 2. cathartic Acute anxiety: 1. IV or PO diazepam Psychological and supportive care	LSD is available on the street in the form of tablets, capsules, sugar cubes, or solution on blotting paper ("blotter acid" or "postage stamps"). Street name includes "California sunshine." A quiet, nonthreatening environment may be helpful in "talking down" patients. Trauma as result of altered behavior may be noted.
Barbiturates Short acting: 1. Pentobarbital 2. Butalbital Long acting: 1. Phenobarbital 2. Primidone	Neurologic: CNS depression, including coma CV: hypotension, cardiovascular collapse	Plasma levels (serial)	Supportive care: 1. airway 2. breathing 3. circulation	Barbiturates are used as anticonvulsants and sedatives. Drug withdrawal may occur.

	Respiratory: respiratory arrest		Prevention of absorption:
	Temperature regulation: hypothermia		1. lavage
	Dermal: hemorrhagic blisters—"barb burns"		2. activated charcoal (serial)
			3. cathartic
			Specific therapy for phenobarbital:
			1. urine alkalinization
			Symptomatic and supportive care

Carbon Monoxide

Incomplete combustion of carbon-containing fuels	Vital signs: hypotension	Carboxyhemoglobin level	Supportive care:	Carbon monoxide (CO) is the leading cause of poisoning deaths in the United States. CO combines with hemoglobin with an affinity over 200 times greater than that of oxygen. Toxicity results from impaired oxygen delivery and affects primarily the organs most susceptible to hypoxia (heart, brain).
Sources:	CV: myocardial depression, conduction defects	LDH, CPK, SGOT	1. airway	
1. Exhaust from automobiles or any gas engines	Neurologic: headache, lethargy, agitation, confusion, coma, seizures, cerebral edema	Arterial blood gases	2. breathing	
2. Faulty wood/coal stoves	GI: nausea gastroenteritis	CT scan if indicated	3. circulation	
3. Fire	Metabolic: acidosis	Cardiac monitor	100% oxygen through a tight-fitting mask or endotracheal tube if patient lacks adequate ventilation	
4. Methylene chloride found in paint and varnish remover converts to carbon monoxide		Chest radiograph	Hyperbaric oxygen therapy for symptomatic patients	
			Correct acidosis	

(continued)

Commonly Observed Poisonings (continued)

Substance/Examples	Nursing Assessment	Diagnostic	Intervention	Comments
Cyclic Antidepressants				
Amitriptyline Imipramine Desipramine Nortriptyline Trimipramine Doxepin Amoxapine Protriptyline Tetracyclics	Vital signs: tachycardia, hypertension followed by hypotension, respiratory depression CV: ventricular dysrhythmias and conduction block Neurologic: lethargy, coma, seizures, myoclonus GI: decreased bowel sounds, dry mouth, urinary retention	Urine/blood for tricyclics Electrolytes Arterial blood gases Serial 12-lead ECG	Supportive care: 1. airway 2. breathing 3. circulation Prevention of absorption: 1. lavage 2. activated charcoal 3. cathartic Hypotension: fluids, and, if necessary, norepinephrine is the vasopressor of choice Cardiac monitor Seizure precautions Correct acidosis with sodium bicarbonate or hyperventilation on ventilator Correct conduction disturbances with serum alkalinization to a pH of 7.45–7.55 Monitor bowel sounds	Cyclic antidepressants are used in the treatment of endogenous depression. CNS and CV toxicity are the major complications of this overdose. Certain newer compounds such as amoxapine appear to have more CNS than CV affects.

Marijuana	Vital signs: tachycardia, postural hypotension Neurologic: alteration in mood, cognition, motor coordination and heightened sensory awareness, lethargy, euphoria GI: stimulation of appetite, dry mouth, nausea	Urine/plasma screen	Supportive care: 1. airway 2. breathing 3. circulation Prevention of absorption: 1. ipecac 2. charcoal 3. cathartic Benzodiazepines for sedation Calm environment IV fluids and Trendelenburg position for hypotension	The individual response to recreational use of marijuana depends on the dose, the personality and expectations of the user, and the setting. Initial effects range from euphoria and relaxation to paranoia and manic psychosis. Adults usually require only supportive care after overdose. Accidental ingestion by children may require prevention of absorption if seen within 3 hr of exposure.
Opioids	Vital signs: hypotension, bradycardia, decreased respirations, hypothermia CV: bradycardia Neurologic: pinpoint pupils, coma, respiratory depression, seizures	Urine/plasma screen Arterial blood gases	Supportive care: 1. airway 2. breathing 3. circulation Prevention of absorption: 1. lavage 2. charcoal 3. cathartic	An attempt should be made to get a complete history of the overdose, including route of exposure, quantities, and type of drug used, and history of addiction. Monitor in an intensive care facility.

(continued)

Commonly Observed Poisonings (continued)

Substance/Examples	Nursing Assessment	Diagnostic	Intervention	Comments
Opioids (continued)			Cardiac monitor Management of withdrawal Antidote: Naloxone Evaluation for pulmonary edema	
Ethylene Glycol Antifreeze	Neurologic: ataxia, lethargy, coma, seizures GU: calcium oxaluria, hematuria, proteinuria, renal insufficiency Respiratory: pulmonary edema CV: cardiomegaly	Serum ethylene glycol level Electrolytes Arterial blood gases Renal function tests Urinalysis Osmolar gap (use plasma osmolarity measured with freezing point depression method)	Supportive care: 1. airway 2. breathing 3. circulation Prevention of absorption: 1. ipecac 2. lavage 3. activated charcoal 4. cathartic Correction of acidosis with IV sodium bicarbonate	Ethylene glycol toxicity may result in CNS effects similar to those seen with ethanol toxicity. Anion gap metabolic acidosis may result from the production of toxic metabolities. Oxalic acid formation may contribute to renal injury. Supplying ethanol competitively inhibits alcohol dehydrogenase, subsequently impairing the metabolism of ethylene

Ethanol drip:
1. monitor glucose
2. monitor blood alcohol level

Hemodialysis (may be indicated for levels > 50 mg/dl, renal failure, or uncorrected acid–base or electrolyte abnormalities)

Evaluation of renal function

glycol to its toxic metabolic. If IV ethanol is not available, oral ethanol may be given until the IV form is available.

Acetaminophen

Acetaminophen-containing commercial products:

Excedrin Extra Strength Tablet

Liquiprin Tablet

Tempura Chewable Table

Tylenol PM

Phase 1 (up to 24 hr postingestion): anorexia, nausea, vomiting, diaphoresis, malaise

Phase 2 (after 24 hr): RUQ pain, increased liver function tests and total bilirubin

Phase 3 (3–5 days): characterized by sequelae of hepatic necrosis: coagulation defects, jaundice, renal failure, hepatic encephalopathy

Phase 4: recovery

Acetaminophen level at 4 or more hr postingestion

Daily monitoring of SGOT, total bilirubin, blood urea nitrogen, creatinine, and prothrombin time.

Supportive care:
1. airway
2. breathing
3. circulation

Prevention of absorption:
1. ipecac
2. activated charcoal
3. cathartic

Determination of 4 hr postingestion acetaminophen level (plotted on Rumack–Matthew nomogram)

Acetaminophen is an antipyretic and analgesic over-the-counter preparation. It also is a component of many combination products. Indication for n-acetylcysteine (NAC) therapy is determined by plotting the serum level on the Rumack–Matthew nomogram (Fig. 46–1). NAC is most effective if administered within 8 hr postingestion. Oral NAC

(continued)

Commonly Observed Poisonings *(continued)*

Substance/Examples	Nursing Assessment	Diagnostic	Intervention	Comments
Acetaminophen (continued)			Antidote: N-acetylcysteine (NAC, Mucomyst) 1. loading dose: 140 mg/kg po of 20% solution × 1 dose 2. Maintenance dose: 70 mg/kg of 20% solution × 17 doses q4h 3. Dilute doses 3:1 with soft drink or juice Repeat dose if patient vomits within 1 hr of dose; for persisting vomiting, consider an antiemetic or administration of undiluted drug via nasogastric or duodenal tube	is the only approved drug treatment of acetaminophen poisoning in the U.S. Intravenous NAC is investigational in the U.S. Activated charcoal will interfere with NAC; therefore, do not administer the drugs concurrently.
Organophosphates Chlorphyrifos Dursban Malathion Ortho Malathion 50 Insect Spray	1. Muscarinic effects: a. Increased salivation b. increased lacrimination	Plasma pseudocholinesterase and/or red cell acetylcholinesterase	Supportive care: 1. airway 2. breathing 3. circulation	Organophosphates are widely used in agriculture and for home/garden pest control. Rapid-

Parathion

c. sweating
d. vomiting
e. diarrhea
2. Nicotinic effects:
   a. muscle weakness
   b. respiratory paralysis
   c. fasiculations

Prevention of absorption:
1. ipecac
2. activated charcoal
3. cathartic

Dermal decontamination:
1. Repeated washings with soap and water
2. discard leather products
3. protect health care provider from dermal exposure

Assessment of oral secretions (suction prn)

Pulmonary status monitoring:
1. breath sounds
2. chest radiograph

Antidotes:
1. atropine
2. pralidoxime

acting organophosphates such as Tabun, Sarin, and Soman have been developed as nerve gases for chemical warfare. Well absorbed via oral, dermal, or inhalation routes, these agents exhibit their main effects by preventing the breakdown of the neurotransmitter acetylcholine. The acetylcholine accumulates at the synapses and myoneural junctions, leading to a cholinergic crisis. The efficient dermal absorption requires a rigorous skin decontamination. Leather products are difficult to decontaminate; therefore, the patient's leather shoes, watchband, and belt must be discarded. Atropine blocks the effects of excessive acetylcholine if it persists in

(*continued*)

Commonly Observed Poisonings (continued)

Substance/Examples	Nursing Assessment	Diagnostic	Intervention	Comments
Organophosphates (continued)				high enough concentrations. The administration of over 2,000 mg of atropine has been reported to reverse effects of severe poisoning.[3]
Salicylates Aspirin AlkaSeltzer Aspergum Pepto Bismol Sunscreens Liniments Methyl salicylate (oil of wintergreen)	Respiratory: tachypnea, pulmonary edema, respiratory alkalosis GI: nausea, vomiting, hemorrhage Metabolic: fluid and electrolyte disturbances, metabolic acidosis, hyperthermia, hypokalemia, dehydration, fever Neurologic: tinnitus, confusion, lethargy, coma, seizures	Serial salicylate levels Arterial blood gases Electrolytes Complete blood count, prothrombin time, partial thromboplastin time Platelet count Chest radiograph	Supportive care: 1. airway 2. breathing 3. circulation Prevention of absorption: 1. ipecac 2. lavage 3. activated charcoal (serial doses) 4. cathartic Enhancement of excretion: 1. urine alkalinization to pH 7.5–8.0	Salicylates are used as antipyretic, analgesic, antiinflammatory medications. Absorption may be erratic. Large doses may form concretions in stomach and delay absorption and toxicity. At least two salicylate levels are needed to ensure levels are declining and absorption is not continuing. Urine alkalinization may be difficult without adequate serum potassium.

	Signs and Symptoms	Laboratory	Treatment	Comments
	Hematologic: hypothrombinemia, platelet dysfunction CV: tachycardia		Monitor respiratory status Hemodialysis may be indicated	
Methanol Antifreeze Windshield washer solvent Varnish Sterno Wood alcohol	Vital signs: monitor for apnea Neurologic: headache, vertigo, lethargy confusion; coma and seizures may occur in severe cases Ocular: blurred vision, decreased visual acuity, photophobia GI: nausea, vomiting, abdominal pain	Blood methanol Arterial blood gases Electrolytes Anion gap Glucose, blood alcohol while on ethanol drip	Supportive care: 1. airway 2. breathing 3. circulation Prevention of absorption: 1. ipecac/lavage 2. charcoal/cathartic ineffective Antidotes: 1. ethanol drip for blood methanol level greater than 20 mg/dl 2. Folic acid to enhance the metabolism of formic acid Correct acidosis with sodium bicarbonate	Methanol is an alcohol commonly found in antifreeze, windshield washer fluid, and Sterno. Methanol is metabolized to formaldehyde and formic acid, both of which are much more toxic than methanol itself. These two end products produce severe acidosis and blindness, with the onset of symptoms in several hours to several days. The administration of intravenous alcohol is the treatment of choice. Alcohol competes with methanol at the enzyme

(continued)

Commonly Observed Poisonings (continued)

Substance/Examples	Nursing Assessment	Diagnostic	Intervention	Comments

Methanol (continued)			Monitor electrolytes, creatinine, calcium, blood urea nitrogen and serum methanol and ethanol levels
			
			Enhancement of elimination:
			1. Hemodialysis indications:
			  a. Methanol level over 50 mg/dl
			  b. Metabolic acidosis not immediately correctable with bicarbonate therapy.
			  c. Visual impairment
			  d. Renal failure
				site in the liver, blocking the formation of toxic metabolites and allowing methanol to be excreted unchanged. The drip must be continued until the blood methanol level is less than 20 mg/dl and acidosis is corrected.

CNS, central nervous system; CV, cardiovascular; GI, gastrointestinal; HEENT, head, eyes, ear, nose, throat; LDH, lactate dehydrogenase; CPK, creatinine phosphokinase; SGOT, serum glutamic oxaloacetic transaminase; CT, computed tomography; ECG, electrocardiogram; GU, genitourinary; IV, intravenous.

Universal Precautions and Health Care Worker Protection

Because a person's HIV status often is unknown or difficult to ascertain, it is recommended that:

- All patients be treated with universal precautions
- Barriers be used for the protection of both the health care worker and the patient

Potentially Infected Body Fluids

- Blood
- Pleural fluid
- Semen
- Vaginal fluid
- Pericardial fluid
- Peritoneal fluid
- Cerebrospinal fluid
- Synovial fluid
- Amniotic fluid
- Breast milk
- Soft tissue fluid (released on traumatic contact)

Wear Gloves for

- Phlebotomy
- Placing and removing intravenous lines
- Contact with laboratory specimens
- Dressing changes (simple)
- Lumbar punctures

Wear Gloves, Masks, Protective Eyewear for

- Intubation
- Airway manipulation
- Oral procedures

Wear Gloves, Masks, Protective Eyewear, and Gowns for

- Placement of arterial catheters
- Placement of central venous catheters
- Bronchoscopy
- Endoscopy
- Nasal intubation
- Thoracentesis
- Complex wound care
- Dialysis
- Surgery

Factors Predisposing to Specific Aspects of Compromised Host Defenses

Host Defect	Diseases, Therapies and Other Conditions Associated With Host Defects
Impaired phagocyte functioning	Radiation therapy
	Nutritional deficiencies
	Diabetes mellitus
	Acute leukemias
	Corticosteroids
	Cytotoxic chemotherapeutic drugs
	Aplastic anemia
	Congenital hematologic disorders
	Alcoholism
Complement system deficiencies	Liver disease
	Systemic lupus erythematosus
	Sickle cell anemia
	Splenectomy
	Congenital deficiencies
Impaired cell-mediated (T lymphocyte) immune response	Radiation therapy
	Nutritional deficiencies
	Aging
	Thymic aplasia
	AIDS
	Hodgkin's disease/lymphomas
	Corticosteroids
	Antilymphocyte globulin
	Congenital thymic dysfunctions
Impaired humoral (antibody) immunity	Chronic lymphocytic leukemia
	Multiple myeloma
	Congenital hypogammaglobulinemia
	Protein-liosing enteropathies (inflammatory bowel disease)

(*continued*)

**Factors Predisposing to Specific Aspects
of Compromised Host Defenses (continued)**

Host Defect	Diseases, Therapies and Other Conditions Associated With Host Defects
Interruption of physical/mechanical/chemical barriers	Traumatic injury
	Decubitus ulcers/skin defect
	Invasive medical procedures
	Vascular disease
	Skin diseases
	Nutritional impairments
	Burns
	Respiratory intubation
	Mechanical obstruction of body drainage systems such as lacrimal and urinary systems
	Decreased level of consciousness
Impaired reticuloendothelial system	Liver disease
	Splenectomy

From Larson E: Infection control issues in critical care: An update. Heart Lung 14:149–155, 1985.

Overview of the Epidemiology of AIDS

Occurrence	Worldwide and increasing everywhere. Highest in persons with identified risk factors: homosexual and bisexual males, heterosexual contact with persons with AIDS, intravenous drug abuse, transfusion recipients, hemophilia or coagulation disorder, infant born of HIV-positive mother.
Etiologic agent	Human immunodeficiency virus (HIV); two types of HIV virus have been identified: HIV-1 (prevalent in the United States) and HIV-2 (prevalent in West Africa and countries with epidemiologic links to West Africa).
Reservoir	Humans.
Transmission	The virus is present in blood and serum-derived body fluids; transmitted person to person through anal or vaginal intercourse, transplacentally, and by breastfeeding; transmitted indirectly by transfusion of contaminated blood or blood products, use of contaminated needles or syringes, or direct contact with infected blood or body fluids on mucous membranes or open wounds; theoretically possible to transmit by oral/genital contact and deep French kissing. There are no reports of transmission from saliva, tears, urine, bronchial secretions, biting insects or any type of casual contact.
Incubation period	Variable. The time from exposure to seroconversion is 4 weeks to 6 months. The time to symptomatic immune suppression and to AIDS diagnosis can be up to 20 years.
Period of communicability	Lifelong; from presence of HIV in sera until death. The degree of contagiousness may vary during the course of HIV infection.
Susceptibility and resistance	Unknown; presumed to be general. Antibody response is not protective.
Report to local health authority	AIDS case report required. Report of HIV positive status varies by state.

Data from Benensen A (ed): Control of Communicable Diseases in Man, 15th ed. Washington, DC, The American Public Health Association, 1990.
Reproduced by permission from Grimes E: Infectious Diseases. St. Louis, Mosby Year Book, 1991.

1993 Revision of Case Definition for AIDS for Surveillance Purposes

Conditions Included in the 1993 AIDS Surveillance Case Definition

- Candidiasis of bronchi, trachea, or lungs
- Candidiasis, esophageal
- Cervical cancer, invasive*
- Coccidioidomycosis, disseminated or extrapulmonary
- Cryptococcosis, extrapulmonary
- Cryptosporidiosis, chronic intestinal (>1 month's duration)
- Cytomegalovirus disease (other than liver, spleen, or nodes)
- Cytomegalovirus retinitis (with loss of vision)
- Encephalopathy, HIV-related
- Herpes simplex: chronic ulcer(s) (>1 month's duration); or bronchitis, pneumonitis, or esophagitis
- Histoplasmosis, disseminated or extrapulmonary
- Isosporiasis, chronic intestinal (>1 month's duration)
- Kaposi's sarcoma
- Lymphoma, Burkitt's (or equivalent term)
- Lymphoma, immunoblastic (or equivalent term)
- Lymphoma, primary, of brain
- *Mycobacterium avium* complex or *M. kansasii*, disseminated or extrapulmonary
- *Mycobacterium tuberculosis*, any site (pulmonary* or extrapulmonary)
- *Mycobacterium*, other species or unidentified species, disseminated or extrapulmonary
- *Pneumocystis carinii* pneumonia
- Pneumonia, recurrent*
- Progressive multifocal leukoencephalopathy
- *Salmonella* septicemia, recurrent
- Toxoplasmosis of brain
- Wasting syndrome due to HIV
- Also included as an AIDS indicator is a CD4 count of 200 or less cells/μL.

*Added in the 1993 expansion of the AIDS surveillance case definition.

Also included as an AIDS indicator is a CD4 count of 200 or less cell/θL.

From Centers for Disease Control: 1993 Revised Classification System for HIV Infection and Expanded Surveillance Case Definition for AIDS Among Adolescents and Adults. MMWR 41, No. RR-17, December 18, 1992.

Phases of HIV Infection and AIDS

Phase	Length of Phase	Antibodies Detectable	Symptoms	Can be Transmitted
1. Window period	4 wks to 6 mos after infection	No	None	Yes
2. Acute primary HIV infection	1–2 wks	Possible	Flu-like illness	Yes
3. Asymptomatic infection	1–15 or more yrs	Yes	None	Yes
4. Symptomomatic immune suppression	Up to 3 yrs	Yes	Fever, night sweats, weight loss, diarrhea, neuropathy, fatigue, rashes, lymphadenopathy, cognitive slowing, oral lesions	Yes
5. AIDS	Variable: 1–5 yrs from first AIDS-defining condition	Yes	Severe opportunistic infections and tumors in any body system; neurologic manifestations	Yes

From Grimes E: Infectious Diseases. St. Louis, Mosby Year Book, 1991.

Clinical Manifestations of AIDS

Possible Causes	Possible Effects
Oral Manifestations	
Lesions due to: *Candida*, herpes simplex, Kaposi's sarcoma; papillomavirus oral warts; HIV gingivitis or peridontits; oral leukoplakia	Oral pain leading to difficulty in chewing and swallowing, decreased fluid and nutritional intake, dehydration, weight loss and fatigue, disfigurement
Neurologic Manifestations	
AIDS dementia complex due to: direct attack of HIV in nerve cells	Personality changes; impaired cognition, concentration, and judgment; impaired motor ability; weakness; needs assistance with ADL or unable to perform ADL; unable to talk or comprehend; paresis and/or plegia; incontinence; caregiver burden; inability to comply with medical regimen; inability to work; social isolation
Acute encephalopathy due to: therapeutic drug reactions; drug overdose; hypoxia; hypoglycemia from drug-induced pancreatitis; electrolyte imbalance; meningitis or encephalitis resulting from *Cryptococcus*, herpes simplex virus, cytomegalovirus, *Mycobacterium tuberculosis*, syphilis, *Candida, Toxoplasma gondii*; lymphoma; **Cerebral infarction** resulting from: vasculitis, meningovascular syphilis, systemic hypotension, and marantic endocarditis	Headache, malaise, fever; full or partial paralysis; loss of cognitive ability, memory, judgment, orientation or appropriate affect; sensory distortion; seizures, coma, death
Neuropathy due to: inflammatory demyelination resulting from direct HIV attack; drug reactions; Kaposi's sarcoma lesions	Loss of motor control; ataxia; peripheral numbness, tingling, burning sensation; depressed reflexes; inability to work; caregiver burden; social isolation

(continued)

Clinical Manifestations of AIDS *(continued)*

Possible Causes	Possible Effects
Gastrointestinal Manifestations	
Diarrhea due to: *Cryptosporidum, Isospora belli, Microsporidium, Strongyloides stercoides,* cytomegalovirus, herpes simplex, enterovirusus, adenovirus, *Mycobacterium avium intracellulare, Salmonella, Shigella, Campylobacter, Vibrio parahaemolyticus, Candida, Histoplasma capsulatum, Giardia, Entamoeba histolytica,* normal flora overgrowth, lymphoma, and Kaposi's sarcoma	Weight loss, anorexia, fever; dehydration, malabsorption; malaise, weakness and fatigue; loss of ability to perform social functions due to inability to leave house; incontinence and caregiver burden
Hepatitis due to: *Mycobacterium avium intracellulare, Cryptococcus,* cytomegalovirus, *Histoplasma, Coccidiomycosis, Microsporidium,* Epstein–Barr virus, hepatitis A, B, C, D (delta agent) and E viruses, lymphoma, Kaposi's sarcoma, illegal drug use, alcohol abuse, and prescribed drug use (particularly sulfa drugs)	Anorexia, nausea, vomiting, abdominal pain, jaundice; fever, malaise, rash, joint pain, fatigue; hepatomegaly, hepatic failure, death
Biliary dysfunction due to: Cholangitis from cytomegalovirus and *Cryptosporidium;* lymphoma and Kaposi's sarcoma	Abdominal pain, anorexia, nausea, vomiting and jaundice
Anorectal disease due to: perirectal abscesses and fistulas, perianal ulcers and inflammation resulting from infections with *Chlamydia, Lymphogranulum venereum,* gonorrhea, syphilis, *Shigella, Campylobacter, M. tuberculosis,* herpes simplex, cytomegalovirus, *Candida albicans* obstruction from lymphoma; Kaposi's sarcoma and papillomovirus warts	Difficult and painful elimination; rectal pain, itching, diarrhea

Respiratory Manifestations

Infection due to: *Pneumocystis carinii, M. avium intracellulare, M. tuberculosis, Candida, Chlamydia, Histoplasma capsulatum, Toxoplasma gondii, Coccidioides immitis, Cryptococcus neoforms,* cytomegalovirus, influenza viruses, *Pneumococcus, Strongyloides*

Shortness of breath, cough, pain; hypoxia, activity intolerance, fatigue; respiratory failure and death

Lymphoma and Kaposi's sarcoma

Same as above

Dermatologic Manifestations

Staphylococcal skin lesions (bullous impetigo, ecthyma, folliculitis); herpes simplex virus lesions (oral, facial, anal; vulvovaginal); herpes zoster; chronic mycobacterial lesions appearing over lymph nodes or as ulcerations or hemorrhagic macules; other lesions related to infection with *Pseudomonas aeruginosa, Molluscum contagiosum, Candida albicans,* ringworm, *Cryptococcus, Sporotrichosis;* xerosis-induced dermatitis, seborrheic dermatitis; drug reactions (particularly from sulfa-based drugs); lesions from parasites such as scabies or lice; Kaposi's sarcoma; decubiti and impairment in the integrity of the skin resulting from prolonged pressure and incontinence

Pain, itching, burning, secondary infection and sepsis; disfigurement and altered self-image

Sensory System

Vision: Kaposi's sarcoma on conjunctiva or eyelid; cytomegalovirus retinitis

Blindness

Hearing: Acute external otitis and otitis media; hearing loss related to myelopathy, meningitis, cytomegalovirus, and drug reactions

Pain and hearing loss

ADL, activities of daily living.
Reproduced by permission from Grimes, Deanna E.: Infectious Diseases, St. Louis, 1991, Mosby-Year Book, Inc.

Anesthetic Options

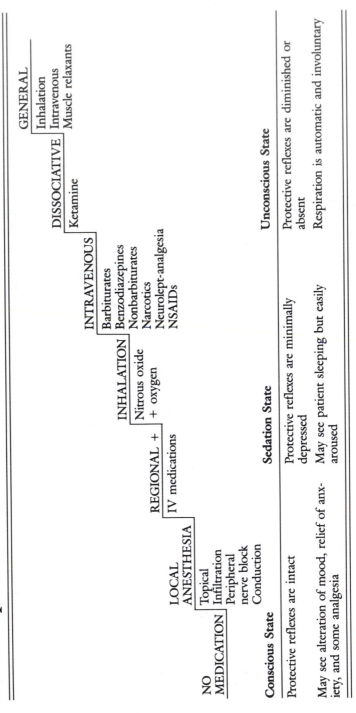

					GENERAL
					Inhalation
					Intravenous
					Muscle relaxants
				DISSOCIATIVE	
				Ketamine	
			INTRAVENOUS		
			Barbiturates		
			Benzodiazepines		
			Nonbarbiturates		
			Narcotics		
			Neurolept-analgesia		
			NSAIDs		
		INHALATION			
		Nitrous oxide + oxygen			
	REGIONAL + IV medications				
LOCAL ANESTHESIA					
Topical					
Infiltration					
Peripheral nerve block					
Conduction					
NO MEDICATION					

Conscious State	Sedation State	Unconscious State
Protective reflexes are intact	Protective reflexes are minimally depressed	Protective reflexes are diminished or absent
May see alteration of mood, relief of anxiety, and some analgesia	May see patient sleeping but easily aroused	Respiration is automatic and involuntary

NSAIDs, nonsteroidal anti-inflammatory drugs; IV, intravenous.

Neuromuscular Blocking Agents

Muscle Relaxants

- Neuromuscular blockers pharmacologically paralyze patients and provide no sedation or analgesia.
- Neuromuscular agents are used to facilitate endotracheal intubation, relax muscles for surgical procedures, terminate laryngospasm, eliminate chest wall rigidity, and for mechanical ventilation if indicated.
- There are two groups of muscle relaxants: depolarizing and nondepolarizing neuroblockers that work at the myoneural junction, affecting the chemical transmitter, acetylcholine.[2, 3]

Depolarizing Agents (Sucostrin, Anectine)

- These drugs combine with acetylcholine receptors at the myoneural junction and mimic the action of acetylcholine.
- Onset of action is 1–2 min and duration of action is 4–6 min.
- The enzyme pseudocholinesterase removes succinylcholine from plasma, so in conditions involving a decrease in pseudocholinesterase, the length of action of succinylcholine increases, keeping patients paralyzed for longer periods.
- Increased pseudocholinesterase enzyme may be seen in pregnancy, liver disease, malnutrition states, severe anemia, cancer, and with other pharmacologic agents such as quinidine, phospholine eye drops, and propranolol.

Nondepolarizing Agents

- Nondepolarizing agents (atacurium, mivacurium chloride, pipecuronium bromide, vecuronium, *d*-tubocurarine, metocurine, pancuronium) compete with acetylcholine at the myoneural junction for muscle membrane receptors.
- Onset of action is within 2–3 min.
- Duration of action ranges from 20 min to 2 hr, depending on the medication and dosage.
- May be reversed pharmacologically with anticholinesterase drugs (neostigmine, pyridostigmine, edrophonium). Duration of action of anticholinesterase is brief, so there is a chance the patient may have continued muscle weakness or respiratory depression. Anticholinesterases may induce muscarinic side effects, including bradycardia, increased salivary, and bronchial secretions. These side effects are counteracted with the routine administration of anticholinergic drugs (atropine, glycopyrrolate) in conjunction with the anticholinesterase.

Medication Choices for Anesthetic Options

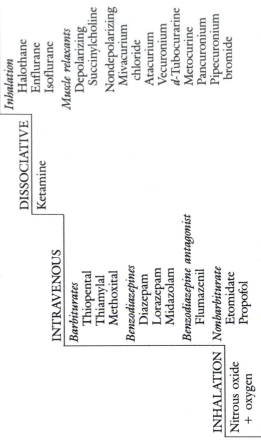

INHALATION
Nitrous oxide
  + oxygen

INTRAVENOUS
Barbiturates
  Thiopental
  Thiamylal
  Methoxital
Benzodiazepines
  Diazepam
  Lorazepam
  Midazolam
Benzodiazepine antagonist
  Flumazenil
Nonbarbiturate
  Etomidate
  Propofol

DISSOCIATIVE
Ketamine

GENERAL
Inhalation
  Halothane
  Enflurane
  Isoflurane
Muscle relaxants
  Depolarizing
    Succinylcholine
  Nondepolarizing
    Mivacurium
      chloride
    Atacurium
    Vecuronium
    d-Tubocurarine
    Metocurine
    Pancuronium
    Pipecuronium
      bromide

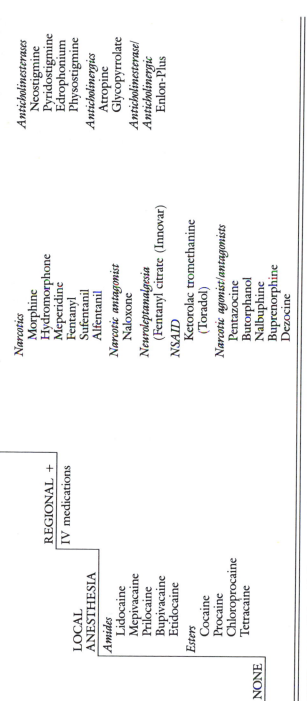

LOCAL ANESTHESIA

Amides
Lidocaine
Mepivacaine
Prilocaine
Bupivacaine
Etidocaine

Esters
Cocaine
Procaine
Chloroprocaine
Tetracaine

REGIONAL +
IV medications

NONE

Narcotics
Morphine
Hydromorphone
Meperidine
Fentanyl
Sufentanil
Alfentanil

Narcotic antagonist
Naloxone

Neuroleptanalgesia
(Fentanyl citrate (Innovar))

NSAID
Ketorolac tromethanine
(Toradol)

Narcotic agonist/antagonists
Pentazocine
Butorphanol
Nalbuphine
Buprenorphine
Dezocine

Anticholinesterases
Neostigmine
Pyridostigmine
Edrophonium
Physostigmine

Anticholinergics
Atropine
Glycopyrrolate

*Anticholinesterase/
Anticholinergic*
Enlon-Plus

NSAID, nonsteroidal anti-inflammatory drugs.

Muscle Relaxant Comparison

	Succinyl-choline	Miva-curium Chloride	Atacurium	Vecuronium	d-Tubo-curarine	Meto-curine	Pancuro-nium	Pipecur-onium Bromide
Onset of action	Within 1–2 min	2–2.5 min	Within 2 min	Within 3 min	Within 3 min	Within 4 min	Within 4 min	5 min
Duration of action	4–6 min	10–15 min	30–45 min	30–40 min	45–60 min	> 60 min	1–1½ hr	1–2 hr
Dose	1 mg/kg	0.10–0.25 mg/kg	0.4–0.5 mg/kg	0.75–1 mg/kg	up to 0.6 mg/kg	0.2 mg/kg	0.04–0.1 mg/kg	0.07–0.85 mg/kg
Metabolism elimination	Enzyme pseudocholinesterase	Plasmacholinesterase Renal and biliary path	Hoffman elimination and ester hydrolysis	Hepatic and renal function	Kidney and liver	Kidney and liver	Kidney and liver	Eliminated by kidneys
Histamine release	Possible	Yes	Mild	Very mild	Yes, causing hypotension and bradycardia	Yes, causing hypotension	Isolated cases	Yes

	Short acting	Intermediate acting		Long acting		
Side effects	↓ Pulse fasciculation Cardiac dysrhythmias Hyperkalemia ↑ ICP ↑ Intraocular pressure	Flushing, hypotension, dysrhythmia, rash, bronchospasm, muscle spasms	Histamine-like reactions	↓ BP	Avoid with myasthenia gravis, true renal disease, hypersensitivity to bromide	Hypertension, atrial fibriliation, CVA, hypoglycemia, hyperkalemia, CNS depressant, respiratory depressant
Advantages	Use with continuous drip; no refrigeration	Little or no cardiovascular effect Easily reversed Block not prolonged	Little or no cardiovascular effect Easily reversed	Useful if cardiovascular disease and hypertension present		Does not cause increased heart rate

Short acting · Intermediate acting · Long acting

Short acting · Intermediate acting · Long acting

ICP, intracranial pressure; CVA, cerebro vascular accident; CNS, central nervous system.

Cardiac Dysrhythmias Associated With Anesthetic Options

Anesthetic Option	Dysrhythmia
Local anesthesia with epinephrine	Tachycardia
Spinal and epidural	Bradycardia 2° vagal response; PACs, PVCs, supraventricular tachycardia, atrial fibrillation 2° sympathetic stimulation; wandering pacemaker and heart block 2° increased vagal tone.
Barbiturates	
Pentothal	Bradycardia, AV dissociation, occasional PVC
Nonbarbiturate etomidate	Sinus tachycardia
Narcotics	
Morphine sulfate	Transient bradycardia
Meperidine hydrochloride	Transient tachycardia
Fentanyl	Bradycardia
Narcotic antagonist	PVCs, ventricular tachycardia, occasional ventricular fibrillation
Neuroleptanalgesia (droperidol component)	Tachycardia
Dissociative agent	Myocardial depression, ventricular ectopy, tachycardia
Inhalation agents	
Halothane	AV dissociation, ventricular dysrhythmias if hypercarbia occurs
Halothane plus aminophylline, cocaine, lidocaine	Bradycardia
Halothane plus pancuronium	PACs and PVCs
Isoflurane	Tachycardia
Enflurane	AV dissociation
Muscle relaxants	
Succinylcholine	Sinus bradycardia, junctional rhythms, PVCs. Patients with burns, trauma, paraplegia or quadriplegia prone to ST depression, peaked T waves, widening QRS leading to ventricular tachycardia, ventricular fibrillation, or asystole
Pipecuronium bromide	Atrial fibrillation, ventricular extrasystole
Pancuronium	Tachycardia and nodal rhythms
d-Tubocurarine	Tachycardia

(*continued*)

Cardiac Dysrhythmias Associated With Anesthetic Options (*continued*)

Anesthetic Option	Dysrhythmia
Anticholinesterases	Bradycardia, slowed AV conduction, PVC
Anticholinergics	Tachycardia

PAC, premature atrial contraction; PVC, premature ventricular contraction; AV, atrioventricular.

Conditions and Medications That Increase the Effects of Nondepolarizing Muscle Relaxants

Local anesthetics
General anesthetics
Antibiotics: aminoglycosides, polypeptides, Polymyxin
Antiarrhythmics: quinidine, procainamide
Furosemide
Acid–base status: respiratory acidosis, metabolic alkalosis
Electrolyte imbalance: hypokalemia, hypocalcemia, dehydration, magnesium administration
Hypothermia

Conditions That Precipitate Dysrhythmias

Hypoxemia
Sinus bradycardia, sinus tachycardia, PVCs, supraventricular tachycardia

Hypoventilation
Sinus tachycardia, PVCs, sinus bradycardia

Hypovolemia
Sinus tachycardia

Fluid overload
PVCs, supraventricular tachycardia, PACs, atrial fibrillation/flutter

Hyperthermia
Sinus tachycardia, PVCs

Pain
Sinus tachycardia, PVCs

Factors Influencing Pain

Surgical procedure: Site and nature of the operation
Anxiety level: Fear of surgery, disfigurement, death, loss of control
Patient expectations: Effectiveness of preoperative teaching, adequately prepared for outcome
Pain tolerance: Prior use of medications including analgesics, individual differences
Anesthesia technique: Analgesics used during the intraoperative period, use of naloxone

Hypotension Etiologies

Anesthetic Agents

Regional agents
Narcotics
Tranquilizers
Barbiturates
Muscle relaxants
Inhalation agents

Decreased Venous Return

Hypovolemia
  Inadequate replacement
  Continued blood loss
Hypothermia
Myocardial depression
Third spacing
Sepsis
Transfusion reaction
Tight abdominal dressing
Increased intrathoracic pressure

Cardiac

Dysrhythmias
  Supraventricular tachycardia
Myocardial infarction
Congestive heart failure

Pulmonary

Hypoxia
Acidosis
Pulmonary embolism
Pneumothorax

Vasovagal Reactions

Bradycardia
Pain
Bladder/abdominal distention

Technical Problems

Blood pressure cuff size and position
Transducer balance and calibration
Stethoscope position

Management of Side Effects From Epidural Analgesia

Specific protocols for epidural management are essential for each individual hospital

Urinary retention
    Catheterization may be needed

Postural hypotension
    Fluid (volume) replacement
    Ephedrine 5 mg IV

Pruritus (itching of face, head, and neck)
    Treat with benadryl 25 mg PO, IM, IV
    Treat with naloxone 01. mg IV

Nausea and vomiting
    Metoclopramide 10 mg IV
    Droperidol 0.25 mg IV
    Scopolamine patch

Respiratory depression (risk increases with age)
    First signs may be change in level of consciousness
    May occur up to 24 hr after narcotic injection with naloxone 0.1 mg up to
    a maximum of 0.4 mg IV
        Continuous observation is imperative because naloxone's duration is 30
        min

Naloxone and ephedrine should be available at the bedside of patients who have received epidural narcotics or anesthetics.

PO, orally; IM, intramuscularly; IV, intravenously.

CHAPTER 10
Nursing Care Plans

Cardiovascular System

Respiratory System

Renal System

Nervous System

Gastrointestinal System

Endocrine System

Hudak: HANDBOOK OF CRITICAL CARE NURSING.
© 1994 J. B. Lippincott Company.

Multisystem Conditions

Cardiac Surgery and Heart Transplantation

NURSING DIAGNOSIS	OUTCOME CRITERIA/ PATIENT GOALS	NURSING ORDERS/INTERVENTIONS
Decreased cardiac output: related to changes in left ventricular preload, afterload, and contractility.	• Hemodynamic stability: BP, CO, PCWP, LAPM, SVR, and LVSWI and SvO₂ will be within patient's normal limits.	1. Maintain arterial, thermodilution and LAP lines.
		2. Assess hemodynamic parameters, including BP, PCWP, LAPM and SVO₂ continuously, and CO, SVR, LVSWI every 1–2 hours.
		3. Administer volume as ordered to optimize PCWP or LAPM.
		4. Administer nitroprusside or other vasodilators as ordered to decrease a high SVR.
		5. Administer positive inotropic agents as ordered to optimize LVSWI. Posttransplant use isoproterenol.
		6. Administer vasopressors as ordered for hypotension <90 mm Hg systolic.

(continued)

***Cardiac Surgery and Heart Transplantation* (*continued*)**

NURSING DIAGNOSIS	OUTCOME CRITERIA/ PATIENT GOALS	NURSING ORDERS/INTERVENTIONS
		7. Assess core body temperature and if lower than 37°C increase room temperature and apply blankets and radiant heat. Warm slowly to prevent shivering or rapid vasodilation.
		8. Maintain normal pH and ABGs.
Decreased cardiac output: related to right ventricular failure, post transplant.	• CVP and pulmonary vascular resistance will be within patient's normal limits.	1. Assess CVP.
		2. Calculate pulmonary vascular resistance.
		3. Administer isoproterenol or other vasodilator to decrease elevated pulmonary vascular resistance.
Decreased cardiac output: related to acute rejection.	• Rejection will be prevented.	1. Administer immunosuppressive medications, as ordered.
		2. Monitor cyclosporine trough levels.
		3. Prepare patient for endomyocardial biopsy.
Decreased cardiac output: related to dysrhythmias or conduction disturbances.	• Cardiac rate and rhythm will be adequate to maintain systemic perfusion.	1. Monitor cardiac rate and rhythm continuously.
		2. Document rhythm strip every shift and with any change.

Decreased cardiac output: related to dysrhythmias in the denervated heart post transplant.

- Sinus mechanism will be maintained between 90 and 110 beats/min.

3. Assess BP and apical and radial pulse.
4. If temporary pacemaker is in use, assess proper functioning including rate, capture, sensing, and settings; maintain electrical safety.
5. Maintain normal electrolyte levels—especially potassium.
6. Maintain adequate ABGs.
7. Administer antiarrhythmics, as ordered.
8. Relieve anxiety or pain which can aggravate dysrhythmias.
9. Obtain 12-lead ECG.
1. Administer isoproterenol or use pacemaker as ordered for brady-arrhythmias—not atropine.
2. Use β-blockers, Ca^+ channel blockers, or cardioversion as ordered for SVT—not vagal maneuvers or digitalis.

Fluid volume deficit: related to increased capillary permeability with fluid shift from intravascular to interstitial space.

- Intravascular volume will be sufficient to maintain adequate cardiac output.

1. Assess BP, CVP, PCWP, LAPM continuously.
2. Administer crystalloids, colloids, or blood as ordered.

(continued)

Cardiac Surgery and Heart Transplantation (continued)

NURSING DIAGNOSIS	OUTCOME CRITERIA/ PATIENT GOALS	NURSING ORDERS/ INTERVENTIONS
		3. Measure input and output.
		4. Autotransfuse chest tube drainage according to unit protocol.
Fluid volume excess: related to hemodilution, increased vasopressin, and aldosterone levels.	• Adequate urine output will be maintained.	1. Assess CVP, PCWP, LAPM continuously.
		2. Assess for peripheral edema.
		3. Measure input and output.
		4. Weigh patient daily.
		5. Administer mannitol, Lasix or other diuretic, as ordered.
		6. Implement fluid restriction, as ordered.
		7. Maintain sodium restriction, as ordered.
Altered tissue perfusion: related to cardiopulmonary bypass, decreased cardiac output, hypotension.	• Systolic BP will be maintain between 90 and 150 mm Hg and SvO₂ between 60% and 80%.	1. Assess BP, hemodynamic parameters, and SvO₂.
	• Peripheral pulses will be palpable.	2. Assess skin and peripheral pulses.
	• Return of preoperative mental status.	3. Implement measures to optimize cardiac output.
		4. Administer vasopressors, as ordered.

5. Assess neurological status including pupillary reaction, level of consciousness, and response to commands initially, hourly, and whenever a change is noted until the patient is fully recovered from anesthesia.

Altered tissue perfusion: related to denervation of the donor heart post transplant.

- Patient will have no episodes of postural hypotension.

1. Instruct patient to change position slowly.
2. Instruct patient to warm up and cool down over prolonged period with exercise.

Impaired gas exchange: related to cardio-pulmonary bypass, anesthesia, poor chest expansion, atelectasis, retained secretions.

- SaO$_2$ and SvO$_2$ will remain within normal limits.

1. Assess rate and depth of respiration.
2. Auscultate breath sounds.
3. Maintain patent airway and integrity of ET tube and ventilator.
4. Monitor SaO$_2$ and SvO$_2$ continuously.
5. Obtain chest x-ray.
6. Obtain ABGs.
7. Adjust tidal volume, FiO$_2$ and respiratory rate as ordered to optimize blood gases.
8. Apply PEEP as ordered to improve oxygenation. Observe for decreased BP and CO as a result of PEEP.

(continued)

Cardiac Surgery and Heart Transplantation (continued)

NURSING DIAGNOSIS	OUTCOME CRITERIA/PATIENT GOALS	NURSING ORDERS/INTERVENTIONS
		9. Suction as needed and observe amount, color, and consistency of secretions.
		10. Extubate as ordered when patient is alert and extubation criteria are met.
		11. After extubation: administer oxygen; cough, deep breathe q1–2h initially then q2–4h; assist with incentive spirometry q2h; advance activity as tolerated.
		12. Teach patient how to splint median sternotomy incision.
		13. Administer analgesics to facilitate coughing and incentive spirometry.
Alterations in comfort: related to ET tube, surgical incisions, chest tubes, rib spreading.	• Patient will verbalize relief from pain, appear comfortable, and be able to rest.	1. Assess character, location, intensity, and duration of pain.
		2. Differentiate between pain from the median sternotomy and pain from angina.
		3. Position for comfort and provide comfort measures such as back rubs.

High risk for anxiety: related to fear of death, surgery, critical care unit environment, recovery process.

4. Teach patient to splint median sternotomy incision.
5. Alleviate factors which enhance pain perception such as fatigue and anxiety.
6. Administer analgesics, as ordered.

- Anxiety will be reduced; patient will appear relaxed without presence of physiological responses to anxiety.

1. Implement preoperative teaching.
2. Orient patient to time and place while awakening and inform that surgery is completed.
3. Assess anxiety level and physiological responses to anxiety such as increased BP and heart rate.
4. Establish trusting, confident relationship with patient and family.
5. Allow patient and family to verbalize feelings and fears.
6. Reassure patient and identify examples of progress (eg, extubation).
7. Provide opportunity for patient and family to participate in care.
8. Administer sedatives as ordered.

High risk for fluid volume deficit: related to abnormal bleeding.

- Chest tube drainage will be less than 100 cc/h.

1. Assess character, amount, and trend of chest tube drainage hourly.

(continued)

Cardiac Surgery and Heart Transplantation (continued)

NURSING DIAGNOSIS	OUTCOME CRITERIA/ PATIENT GOALS	NURSING ORDERS / INTERVENTIONS
		2. Maintain chest tube patency by milking or stripping as needed.
		3. Maintain systolic blood pressure below 150 mm Hg.
		4. Autotransfuse chest drainage according to unit protocol.
		5. Apply PEEP as ordered.
		6. Obtain Hgb and Hct.
		7. Administer volume expanders or blood as ordered to maintain adequate PCWP or LAPM.
		8. Obtain ACT, PT, PTT, bleeding time, platelet count, and fibrinogen levels as ordered.
		9. Administer protamine, platelets, FFP as ordered.
High risk for decreased cardiac output: related to cardiac tamponade.	• Patient will have no evidence of cardiac tamponade.	1. Assess for decreasing BP and increasing and equalizing CVP and PCWP.
		2. Assess for paradoxical pulse >10 mg Hg.

3. Assess patency of chest tubes and for abrupt decrease in amount of drainage.

4. Milk or strip chest tubes to restore patency.

5. Administer fluids or vasopressors as ordered to maintain CO and BP.

6. Obtain chest x-ray as ordered.

7. Anticipate patient's return to OR.

High risk for infection: related to surgical procedure, invasive lines, drainage tubes, hypoventilation, retained secretions, or immunosuppression for post transplant patients.

- Patient will be free from postoperative infections.

1. Assess incisions and all invasive lines and tubes daily for erythema, swelling, and drainage.

2. Assess temperature q4h.

3. Discontinue invasive lines and drainage tubes as soon as possible.

4. Keep incisions clean and dry.

5. Administer prophylactic antibiotics as ordered.

6. Assess breath sounds q4h.

7. Assist patient to cough and use incentive spirometer q2h.

8. Observe character and consistency of sputum.

(continued)

Cardiac Surgery and Heart Transplantation (continued)

NURSING DIAGNOSIS	OUTCOME CRITERIA/ PATIENT GOALS	NURSING ORDERS/INTERVENTIONS
	• The post transplant patient will not develop postoperative infections.	9. Increase activity level as tolerated.
		10. Implement private room and meticulous handwashing or protective isolation per unit protocol.
		11. Report any temperature elevation.
		12. Obtain cultures of wounds, urine, sputum as ordered.
		13. Administer mycostatin oral rinse as ordered.
		14. Monitor cyclosporine and leukocyte levels.
		15. Use strict aseptic technique when caring for all incisions and insertion sites.
High risk for alterations in pattern of urinary elimination: related to hemodilution, cardiopulmonary bypass, decreased cardiac output, renal failure, post transplant cyclosporine nephrotoxicity.	• Urine output will be within acceptable limits.	1. Measure urine output hourly.
		2. Obtain urine specific gravity q4h.
		3. Observe for hematuria.
		4. Maintain adequate cardiac output, BP, and intravascular fluid volume.

5. Administer mannitol, Lasix or other diuretic as ordered.

6. Administer renal dose dopamine as ordered.

7. Assess BUN, creatinine, and cyclosporine trough levels and notify physician if elevated.

High risk for anxiety: related to critical illness, fear of death or disfigurement, role changes within social setting, or permanent disability.

- Patient will be able to express anxieties to appropriate resource person.

1. Provide environment that encourages open discussion of emotional issues.

2. Mobilize patient's support system and involve these resources as appropriate.

3. Allow time for patient to express self.

4. Identify possible hospital resources for patient/family support.

5. Encourage open family–nurse communications regarding emotional issues.

6. Validate patient and family knowledge base regarding the critical illness.

7. Involve religious support systems as appropriate.

The Patient Undergoing IABP Therapy

NURSING DIAGNOSIS	OUTCOME CRITERIA/ PATIENT GOALS	NURSING ORDERS/INTERVENTIONS
High risk for decreased cardiac output: related to improper or ineffective IABP timing.	• Maintenance of hemodynamic stability as demonstrated by proper waveforms.	1. Place assist ratio on 1:2 and verify correct IABP timing hourly.
		2. Document IABP settings hourly to illustrate trends and improvement.
		3. Reevaluate timing for any increase or decrease in heart rate greater than 10 beats/min.
		4. Maintain proper balloon volume.
		5. Refill balloon every 2–4 hr as needed. Use automatic filling mode if available.
		6. Maintain good arterial waveform to allow for evaluation of timing. Notify physician if line starts to fail so a new line can be inserted.
		7. Reduce or eliminate situations which will interfere with the IABPs ability to maintain proper assist ratio. • Maintain adequate ECG signal.

- Alert physician if irregular heart rhythms or rapid tachycardias occur.
  - Initiate pacing or antiarrhythmic drug therapy as ordered.
8. Avoid flexion of hip, which may impair gas movement in and out of IABP catheter.

High risk for altered peripheral perfusion: decreased related to impaired circulation in lower extremity related to presence of catheter, emboli, or thrombosis.

- Patient will have palpable peripheral pulses with skin that is warm, dry, and of normal color.

1. Document quality of peripheral pulses before IABP insertion.
2. Assess peripheral pulses, skin temperature, and color hourly and document.
3. Notify physician of any decrease in pulses.
4. Maintain anticoagulation at prescribed level.
5. Maintain head of bed at a 15° angle or lower to avoid hip flexion, which might obstruct distal flow in the cannulated leg.
6. Maintain cannulated leg in a straight position to avoid hip flexion. Restrain or brace as needed.
7. Maintain balloon motion to prevent thrombus formation on balloon.

(*continued*)

The Patient Undergoing IABP Therapy (continued)

NURSING DIAGNOSIS	OUTCOME CRITERIA/ PATIENT GOALS	NURSING ORDERS/INTERVENTIONS
		8. Assist patient with ankle flexion and extension hourly to promote venous return and prevent venous stasis and potential deep venous thrombosis.
		9. Immediately evaluate peripheral perfusion with any complaints of leg/foot pain by patient.
High risk for impaired gas exchange: related to immobility, sedation, and secretions.	• Oxygenation will be normal, as evidenced by arterial blood gases.	1. Auscultate breath sounds every 2–4 hr and document.
		2. Assist patient with clearing of secretions by coughing or suctioning as indicated.
		3. If intubated, suction at least every 2 hr.
		4. Turn patient every 2 hr.
		5. Obtain order for pulse oximetry if patient has abnormal blood gases, excessive secretions, or respiratory difficulty.

High risk for sensory–perceptual alterations: sensory overload related to critical care unit environment.

• Patient will maintain orientation to name, time, and date and will be able to communicate appropriately.

1. Maintain alarm volumes and monitor noise to lowest possible levels.
2. Minimize unnecessary noise in patient's room.
3. Talk with patient frequently and inform of time and date.
4. Encourage family visits.
5. Explain all procedures, noises, and activities so that patient interprets them appropriately.

High risk for impaired skin integrity: related to immobility, debilitated condition, and impaired circulation.

• Maintenance of normal skin integrity.

1. Assess skin integrity every 2–4 hr and document any redness or ulcerations over bony prominences.
2. Elevate any edematous extremities (only slightly if cannulated extremity is involved).
3. Place sheepskin or foam pad over mattress. Obtain order for air–fluid bed if needed.
4. Turn patient every 2 hr.
5. Massage and lubricate skin exposed to pressure with each repositioning.

(continued)

The Patient Undergoing IABP Therapy (continued)

NURSING DIAGNOSIS	OUTCOME CRITERIA/ PATIENT GOALS	NURSING ORDERS/INTERVENTIONS
		6. Ensure that skin remains clean and dry.
		7. Maintain adequate nutrition by obtaining order for hyperalimentation or nasogastric feedings.
High risk for sleep pattern disturbance: related to critical illness, procedures, and constant monitoring of physiological parameters.	• Patient will have planned blocks of time for undisturbed sleep.	1. Turn down lights in the room during night.
		2. Organize care to allow for progressive increases in uninterrupted time for sleep during night. Amount to be determined by patient condition.
		3. Sedation given patient, as ordered by physician.
High risk for infection: related to a number of indwelling catheters and debilitated condition.	• Patient will remain afebrile, with a normal white blood cell count and negative cultures.	1. Monitor and record temperature every 2 hr.
		2. Observe all insertion sites and incisions daily for signs of infection with dressing changes.
		3. Report any elevation of white blood cell count to physician.

4. Maintain sterile technique with dressing changes.

5. Change any dressing that becomes wet or is not intact.

6. Change all infusion lines, stopcocks, and infusions as per unit protocol.

7. Culture any site with suspicious drainage, redness, or swelling.

8. Give antibiotic, as ordered by physician.

The Patient With Acute Myocardial Infarction

NURSING DIAGNOSIS	OUTCOME CRITERIA/ PATIENT GOALS	NURSING ORDERS/INTERVENTIONS
Alteration in comfort: chest pain related to angina, MI	• Patient will have relief from chest pain.	1. Administer pain medication (nitrates or narcotics) as ordered. 2. Assess relief of pain (using the scale of 1–10). 3. Instruct the patient to notify staff of further pain. 4. Minimize MvO_2; encourage bed rest; provide quiet environment, easily digestible meals, stool softeners. 5. Obtain 12-lead ECG as ordered. 6. Assess history: onset location, duration description, severity of pain (using the scale of 1–10), radiation, precipitating events. 7. Initiate or maintain IV line and oxygen (2–4 L/min).
Decreased cardiac output: electrical factors affecting rate, rhythm, or conduction	• Maintain a cardiac rhythm with adequate systemic perfusion.	1. Conduct continuous cardiac monitoring in MCL_1 or lead II. 2. Document rhythm strip during every shift and as changes in rhythm occur.

Decreased cardiac output: mechanical factors relating to preload, afterload, left ventricular failure

• Maintain hemodynamic stability.

3. Assess BP, apical/radial pulse for extrasystoles, perfusion of extrasystoles.

4. Administer antiarrhythmics, as ordered.

5. Check skin color, temperature.

6. Obtain 12-lead ECG, as ordered.

1. Assess BP, dyspnea, level of consciousness, hypoxemia, tachypnea, orthopnea, crackles, S_3 ventricular gallop, jugular vein distention, urine output, daily weight, peripheral edema, skin color, and temperature.

2. Maintain IV line, intake and output, oxygen, and bed rest.

3. Assess hemodynamic parameters: PCWP, CO, and CI.

4. Give medication as ordered: diuretics, crystalloid fluids, nitrates, vasopressors, inotropic agents, afterload reducers.

5. Assess blood gases.

6. Monitor cardiac rhythm.

7. Assess electrolyte balance, especially serum potassium.

(continued)

The Patient With Acute Myocardial Infarction *(continued)*

NURSING DIAGNOSIS	OUTCOME CRITERIA/ PATIENT GOALS	NURSING ORDERS/INTERVENTIONS
		8. Minimize hypoxemia, acidosis, dysrhythmias, pain.
		9. Assess anxiety level of patient and family; instruct and inform at the appropriate level.
		10. If needed, prepare for IABP.
Knowledge deficit: related to illness and impact on patient's future	• Patient will comply with ADL limitations.	1. Initiate nurse–patient relationship that encourages questioning and uses both formal and informal styles.
		2. Include family in care and teaching.
		3. Begin cardiac rehabilitation education: risk factors, pathophysiology, when to seek medical attention, medications, progressive ADL, diet, sexual activity, returning to work, stress reduction.
	• Patient will ask pertinent questions.	4. Evaluate patient's understanding; document teaching and patient's response on the record.
Anxiety: stress related to fear of illness/death and critical care environment	• Patient will recognize and express concerns and fears.	1. Explain environment, all procedures, expectations and equipment.

2. Allow patient free expression.
3. Maximize patient's control of ADL.
4. Include family in patient's care.
5. Assess for normal grieving process: anger, denial, depression, acceptance.
6. Sedate as needed if ordered by physician.
7. Maximize effective coping styles.
8. Document patient's emotional response to critical illness.

• Patient will use effective coping mechanisms.

9. Spend quiet time with patient so that feelings and fears may be explored.

• Patient will demonstrate reduction in fear and anxiety.

High risk for altered tissue perfusion: thrombolytic therapy impact on myocardial tissue

• Patient will have relief of chest pain.

1. Assess all recurring chest pain: onset, location, duration, description, severity (using scale of 1–10) radiation, precipitating factors.
2. Initiate three peripheral IV sites and O₂ (2–4 L/min).
3. Administer IV NTG, as ordered.

(continued)

The Patient With Acute Myocardial Infarction (continued)

NURSING DIAGNOSIS	OUTCOME CRITERIA/ PATIENT GOALS	NURSING ORDERS/ INTERVENTIONS
		4. Assess pain relief (using 1–10 scale).
		5. Instruct patient to inform staff of further pain.
		6. Minimize MvO_2 with restful environment.
		7. Obtain 12-lead ECG, as ordered.
	• Maintain a cardiac rhythm with adequate perfusion.	8. Conduct continuous cardiac monitoring in MCL_1 or lead II.
		9. Document all changes in rhythm with a rhythm strip.
		10. Assess rhythm for AIVR, AV block, or VT.
		11. Assess hemodynamic tolerance of all rhythms.
		12. Administer antiarrhythmics, as ordered.
	• Patient will have minimal bleeding.	13. Assess neurologic, GU, and GI systems hourly while awake, q2h if asleep.

14. Assess occult blood in all secretions/fluids.

15. Assess PTT q2–4h to be 2–2.5 times normal, or as ordered.

16. Gentle oral care; assess gingival bleeding.

17. Provide safe environment to prevent falls, bruising or injury.

18. Assess BP, dyspnea, level of consciousness, hypoxemia, tachycardia, tachypnea, orthopnea, crackles, S_3, JVD, urine output, daily weight, edema, skin color, and temperature.

19. Assess hemodynamic parameters: PCWP, CO, CI; assess blood gases.

20. Monitor cardiac rhythm.

21. Assess all complaints of itching/hives.

22. Administer hydrocortisone 100 mg, IVP, as ordered.

23. Administer Benadryl, 50 mg IVP, as ordered.

- Maintain hemodynamic stability.

- Patient will not experience an allergic reaction.

(*continued*)

The Patient With Acute Myocardial Infarction (continued)

NURSING DIAGNOSIS	OUTCOME CRITERIA/ PATIENT GOALS	NURSING ORDERS/INTERVENTIONS
High risk for alteration in comfort: chest pain related to pericarditis	• Patient will have relief from pain.	1. Assess pain: onset, location, duration, description, severity (using scale of 1–10), radiation, precipitating factors. 2. Determine whether pain increases with deep breathing, presence of friction rub. 3. Assess rhythm, BP, and heart rate during pain. 4. Administer anti-inflammatory agents as ordered. 5. Explain pathology to patient. 6. Assess pain relief (using scale of 1–10).
High risk for decreased cardiac output: profound shock and heart failure related to acute structural changes (septal rupture, papillary muscle rupture, or cardiac muscle rupture)	• Maintain hemodynamic stability.	1. Assess for sudden onset hypotension, systolic murmur, and pulmonary edema. 2. Assess hemodynamic parameters: PCWP, cardiac output, CI. 3. Prepare for IABP support and possible surgery.

4. Administer afterload reducers and vasopressors as ordered.

5. Minimize MvO$_2$: bed rest, supplemental oxygen, NPO, quiet environment.

6. Monitor cardiac rhythm.

7. Provide emotional support and appropriate explanations to patient and family.

1. Provide environment that encourages open discussion of emotional issues.

2. Mobilize patient's support system and involve these resources as appropriate.

3. Allow time for patient to express self.

4. Identify possible hospital resources for patient/family support.

5. Encourage open family-to-nurse communications regarding emotional issues.

6. Validate patient and family knowledge base regarding the critical illness.

7. Involve religious support systems as appropriate.

High risk for anxiety: related to critical illness, fear of death or disfigurement, role changes within social setting or permanent disability

• Patient will express anxieties to appropriate resource person.

The Patient With Adult Respiratory Distress Syndrome

NURSING DIAGNOSIS

Impaired gas exchange: related to refractory hypoxemia and pulmonary interstitial/alveolar leaks found in alveolar capillary injury states.

OUTCOME CRITERIA/ PATIENT GOALS

- Adequate oxygenation.

NURSING ORDERS / INTERVENTIONS

1. Assess breath sounds q2–4h.
2. Assess for signs of respiratory distress: increased heart rate, agitation, diaphoresis, cyanosis.
3. Assess chest excursion/symmetry.
4. Monitor input and output, observing effects of diuresis and fluid administration.
5. Assess rhythm/dysrhythmias by ECG monitoring.
6. Check ABGs for ↓ PaO_2, ↑ $PaCO_2$.
7. Administer and monitor bronchodilator therapy (eg, theophylline and sympathomimetic agents), as ordered.
8. Maintain mechanical ventilation.
9. Follow serial chest radiograph reports.

Ineffective airway clearance: related to increased secretion production and decreased ciliary motion.

- Maintain patent airway.

- Aspiration will not occur

- Secretions will remain liquid and readily cleared.

1. Assess breath sounds q2—4h and prn.
2. Maintain proper position of tracheostomy or endotracheal tube.
3. Suction tracheostomy/endotracheal tube, oral and nasal cavities, using sterile technique. Note color, amount, and consistency of secretions.
4. Postural drainage and chest percussion when appropriate to augment secretion clearance.
5. Position to facilitate good gas exchange q2h.
6. Monitor for signs of respiratory distress.
7. Maintain adequate cuff pressures/minimal leak technique to avoid aspiration of secretions and tissue necrosis.
8. Elevate head of bed during tube feedings.
9. Provide supplemental humidification.
10. Prepare for bronchoscopy, as ordered.

(*continued*)

The Patient With Adult Respiratory Distress Syndrome (continued)

NURSING DIAGNOSIS	OUTCOME CRITERIA/ PATIENT GOALS	NURSING ORDERS/INTERVENTIONS
Fluid volume excess: related to noncardiac pulmonary edema, PEEP causing a decreased venous return/cardiac output, or diuretic therapy.	• Maintain hemodynamic stability.	1. Weigh patient daily. 2. Monitor total input and output q1h. 3. Assess signs and symptoms of decreased cardiac output: elevated pulse, decreased BP, decreased urine output, change in mentation, decreased PCO_2.
		4. Assess signs of fluid overload: dependent edema, increased weight, pulmonary crackles, respiratory distress, increased CVP.
		5. Monitor hemodynamic parameters: MAP, PCWP, and cardiac output. 6. Administer/monitor IV fluid and electrolyte therapy, as ordered.
	• Urine output will be adequate	7. Monitor total input and output q1h. 8. Report urine output <30 ml/hr to physician. 9. Administer diuretics as ordered. 10. Evaluate BUN and serum creatinine as ordered.

Altered tissue perfusion: related to decreased venous return and decreased cardiac output with PEEP therapy, edema from volume overload, hypotension from shock and ventilation/perfusion mismatch, resulting in hypoxemia.

- Patient will be awake and alert.

- Patient will have warm skin and not be diaphoretic.

- Patient will have normal bowel sounds and abdomen will not be tender.

- Maintain adequate distal peripheral pulses.

1. Assess mental status.

2. Allow patient to make some care decisions.

3. Assess for decreased perfusion to skin.

4. Assess hemodynamic status (PAP, PCWP, CVP).

5. Assess ECG rhythm.

6. Assess GI system: bowel sounds, nausea, vomiting, tenderness.

7. Assess nutritional status.

8. Assess dorsalis pedis, posterior tibial, and radial artery pulses for quality q4h.

9. Evaluate capillary refill time.

Ineffective breathing pattern: related to inadequate gas exchange, increased secretions, decreased ability to oxygenate adequately, fear or exhaustion.

- Work of breathing will be minimized by maintaining bed rest or low level ADLs.

1. Monitor meticulously for onset/progress of signs of respiratory distress.

(*continued*)

The Patient With Adult Respiratory Distress Syndrome (continued)

NURSING DIAGNOSIS	OUTCOME CRITERIA/ PATIENT GOALS	NURSING ORDERS/INTERVENTIONS
		2. Position to facilitate breathing, usually with head of bed elevated.
		3. Reassure patient by confident and calming approach. Stay with patient.
		4. Review serial radiograph reports.
		5. Monitor serial ABGs.
		6. Administer oxygen as indicated.
		7. Use oximetric device to evaluate O_2 saturation during activity.
		8. Sedation, as ordered, prn.
		9. Evaluate all subjective complaints.
		10. Turn, cough, deep breathe q2h.
		11. Suction prn.
		12. Analgesics for pain prn, as ordered.
		13. If patient is ventilated, develop alternate communication system and use soft restraints as needed, if agitated.

High risk for anxiety: related to critical illness, fear of death or disfigurement, role changes within social setting, or permanent disability.

- Patient will be able to express anxieties to appropriate resource person.

1. Establish effective communication with ventilated patient (ie, writing notes).
2. Provide environment that encourages open discussion of emotional issues.
3. Mobilize patient's support system and involve these resources as appropriate.
4. Allow time for patient to express self.
5. Identify possible hospital resources for patient/family support.
6. Encourage open family-to-nurse communications regarding emotional issues.
7. Validate patient and family knowledge base regarding the critical illness.
8. Involve religious support systems as appropriate.

The Mechanically Ventilated Patient

NURSING DIAGNOSIS

Ineffective airway clearance: related to intubation, ventilation, disease process, debilitated state, and fatigue.

OUTCOME CRITERIA/ PATIENT GOALS

• Patient airway will be maintained.

NURSING ORDERS / INTERVENTIONS

1. Auscultate breath sounds q2–4h and prn.

2. Suction only when rhonchi are auscultated (suction pressures should not exceed 100–120 mm Hg). Hyperoxygenate with 4–5 breaths of 100% O_2 and hyperinflate with 1½ times the V_T using a manual resuscitation bag or ventilator. Auscultate breath sounds after suctioning.

3. Monitor ventilator humidifier and temperature (95–100° F).

4. Monitor hydration status of patient to prevent viscous secretions.

5. Monitor dynamic ventilator pressures for sudden increases indicating plugging of airways.

6. Administer saline lavage as indicated for removal of thick secretions.

7. Administer chest physiotherapy as indicated with frequent changes in position.

8. Administer bronchodilator drugs, as ordered, and evaluate their effectiveness on bronchospasms.

9. Turn and position to facilitate gravity drainage of secretions.

Impaired gas exchange: related to retained secretions, disease process, or improper ventilator settings.

• Arterial blood gases will be within normal range for the patient.

1. Obtain ABGs 10–30 min after ventilator changes occur.

2. Monitor ABGs or oximetry during periods of weaning.

3. Assess whether certain positions cause decreased PaO$_2$ or precipitate respiratory discomfort.

4. Monitor for signs and symptoms of hypoxia and hypercapnia.

Ineffective breathing pattern: related to fatigue, improper ventilator settings, increased secretions, or endotracheal tube obstruction.

• Patient will maintain an effective breathing pattern.

1. Perform ventilator checks by qualified nursing personnel or respiratory personnel q1–2h.

2. Evaluate all alarms and determine cause, stat.

3. Maintain a manual resuscitator at the bedside at all times.

(*continued*)

The Mechanically Ventilated Patient (continued)

NURSING DIAGNOSIS	OUTCOME CRITERIA/ PATIENT GOALS	NURSING ORDERS/INTERVENTIONS
		4. Monitor tubing for disconnect, kinking, leaks, or obstruction.
		5. Evaluate cuff pressure/leaks.
		6. Insert a bite block or oral airway to prevent biting on the tube.
		7. Secure endotracheal tube with holder or adhesive tape. Check for breath sounds bilaterally after loosening or changing the tape. Note position at lips in reference to cm markings on the tube.
		8. Position patient to prevent occlusion or dislodging of the tube.
		9. Restrain patient to prevent self-extubation, as per unit protocol.
		10. Evaluate proper positioning of endotracheal tube by x-ray placement and bilateral auscultation.

Altered nutrition, less than body requirements: related to critical illness, increased metabolic needs, lack of ability to consume foods orally.	• Patient will maintain body weight and approach normal weight.	1. Weigh patient daily. 2. Maintain high caloric intake by tube feedings, total parenteral nutrition, and intralipids. Avoid high carbohydrate loads which can elevate $PaCO_2$ levels during weaning. 3. Once trached, evaluate and initiate oral feeding as patient tolerates.
Impaired verbal communication: related to endotracheal tube placement.	• Maintain communication by alternate methods.	1. Explain environment, all procedures, expectations, and equipment. 2. Keep call bell by patient at all times. 3. Provide notepad and pencil, slate, letter or picture board for communication. Ask "yes" or "no" questions. 4. Reassure patient that voice will return once the endotracheal tube is removed. 5. Anticipate and support patient during periods of anxiety and frustration. 6. Remain with patient during process of weaning from ventilator.
Anxiety: related to fear of illness/death and critical care environment; patient and family.	• Patient will use effective coping mechanisms.	1. Maximize patient's control of ADL. 2. Include family in care.

(continued)

The Mechanically Ventilated Patient (continued)

NURSING DIAGNOSIS	OUTCOME CRITERIA/ PATIENT GOALS	NURSING ORDERS/INTERVENTIONS
		3. Sedate as needed if ordered by physician.
		4. Maximize effective coping styles.
		5. Document patient's emotional response to critical illness.
		6. Monitor for signs of ICU psychosis.
		7. Collaborate with physician in providing prognosis and realistic information at patient's level of understanding.
		8. Provide for periods of uninterrupted sleep.
Pain: related to mechanical ventilation, endotracheal tube placement.	• Pain will be relieved or controlled.	1. Maintain tubing position to prevent pulling or jarring of the endotracheal tube.
		2. Adjust ventilator flow rates for comfort.
		3. Adjust ventilator sensitivity to decrease patient's effort to initiate breathing.

4. Position patient with head of bed up unless contraindicated. Change position q2h.

5. Administer analgesic medications as ordered.

High risk for injury: related to mechanical ventilation, endotracheal tube, anxiety, stress.

• Patient will be free from injury during mechanical ventilation.

1. Monitor ventilator for sharp increases on pressure gauge.

2. Observe for signs and symptoms of barotrauma.

3. Monitor cuff pressures q2–4h; maintain cuff pressures 20 mm Hg.

4. Restrain patient to prevent self-extubation.

5. Remove NG ASAP or replace with small feeding tube.

6. Position ventilator tubing to prevent traction on endotracheal tube.

7. Assess endotrachael tube length and document Q shift (ie, "22 cm at tip").

• Patient will not develop stress gastric ulcers.

8. Administer antacids and H$_2$ gastric blockers, as ordered.

9. Sedate patient, as needed.

(continued)

The Mechanically Ventilated Patient *(continued)*

NURSING DIAGNOSIS	OUTCOME CRITERIA/ PATIENT GOALS	NURSING ORDERS/INTERVENTIONS
		10. Monitor patient for abdominal distension, pH of NG aspirate, Hgb and Hct, auscultate bowel sounds, and check stool for occult blood.
High risk for alterations in tissue perfusion: related to positive pressure ventilation, PEEP, hypotension.	• Maintain stable hemodynamics and mentation.	1. Monitor vital signs, PAPs, PCWP, peripheral perfusion, LOC, and input and output.
		2. Perform measurements of hemodynamics with each change in PEEP setting.
		3. Draw mixed venous gases 20 min after each PEEP setting change, as ordered.
		4. Hyperoxygenate/hyperventilate prior to suctioning.
High risk for high risk of infection: related endotracheal tube placement debilitated state.	• Patient will not acquire a nosocomial infection.	1. Evaluate color, amount, consistency, and odor of sputum with each suctioning.
		2. Collect specimens for culture and sensitivity, as indicated.
		3. Maintain sterile technique when suctioning.

4. Change ventilator tubing q24–72h.
5. Perform oral hygiene every shift.
6. Monitor vital signs for indications of infection.
7. Palpate sinuses and visually inspect the tympanic membrane for fevers of unknown origin.
8. Drain condensed water in ventilator tubing externally away from airway and humidifier reservoir.
9. Wash hands frequently.
10. Maintain universal precautions.

1. Monitor ventilator temperature and humidifier q2–4h.
2. Monitor input and output.
3. Weigh patient daily.
4. Calculate lung compliance q2–4h.
5. Monitor serum sodium.
6. Monitor CXR for signs of water retention.
7. Check skin tugor and edema.
8. Auscultate lungs for rales and wheezes q2h.

High risk for alteration in fluid volume excess: related to positive water balance during mechanical ventilation.

• Maintain water balance and normal electrolyte values.

(*continued*)

The Mechanically Ventilated Patient (continued)

NURSING DIAGNOSIS	OUTCOME CRITERIA/ PATIENT GOALS	NURSING ORDERS/INTERVENTIONS
High risk for anxiety: related to critical illness, fear of death or disfigurement, role changes within social setting or permanent disability.	• Patient will be able to express anxieties to appropriate resource person.	1. Provide environment that encourages open expression of emotional issues. 2. Mobilize patient's support system and involve these resources as appropriate. 3. Allow time for patient to express self. 4. Identify possible hospital resources for patient/family support. 5. Encourage open family-to-nurse communications regarding emotional issues. 6. Validate patient and family knowledge base regarding the critical illness. 7. Involve religious support systems as appropriate. 8. Allow patient control over some care, when able.

The Patient With Acute Renal Failure: Prerenal Azotemia

NURSING DIAGNOSIS	OUTCOME CRITERIA/ PATIENT GOALS	NURSING ORDERS/INTERVENTIONS
Altered tissue perfusion: related to hypo-volemia secondary to ARF.	• Patient will be hemodynamically stable.	1. Monitor BP, pulse, respirations, PAP, PCWP, CVP, CO, CI, every hour until stable, then q2h.
		2. Monitor laboratory reports (Na, K, Hgb, Hct, WBC coagulation studies).
		3. Monitor for dry mucous membranes.
		4. Maintain intake and output record.
		5. Daily weights.
		6. Administer fluid and blood per physician's order.
		7. Monitor for fluid overload and/or transfusion reaction.
		8. Weigh patient daily.
		9. Instruct to increase fluid intake to 2,000 ml/day.

(continued)

The Patient With Acute Renal Failure: Prerenal Azotemia (continued)

NURSING DIAGNOSIS	OUTCOME CRITERIA/ PATIENT GOALS	NURSING ORDERS/INTERVENTIONS
		10. Monitor for signs and symptoms of hyponatremia.
		11. Monitor urine output for adequate volume q1h until output is >30 ml/ hr, then take q2h and then q4h.
		12. Test urine for specific gravity every shift. Report abnormalities.
		13. Initiate measures to improve circulation (position changes, maintain warmth).
		14. Monitor temperature and skin color q1h until stable, then q2h.
		15. Monitor for mentation changes (lethargy, stupor).
		16. Reorient to reality frequently. Call by name, tell patient your name, orient to surroundings.

The Patient With Acute Renal Failure: Intrarenal

NURSING DIAGNOSIS	OUTCOME CRITERIA/ PATIENT GOALS	NURSING ORDERS/INTERVENTIONS
Altered tissue perfusion: related to renal ischemia secondary to acute glomerulo-nephritis.	• Patient will maintain fluid and electrolyte balance.	1. Maintain intake and output record. 2. Regulate hydration and avoid dehydration. 3. Observe for signs and symptoms of fluid retention (ie, swelling of ankles). 4. Monitor P, BP, RR. 5. Observe for signs of hyperkalemia; monitor ECG reports. 6. Monitor laboratory values: Na, K, Cl, acid–base balance; administer necessary replacements. 7. Administer Kayexalate as ordered.
High risk for infection: related to ARF.	• Patient will not acquire a nosocomial infection.	1. Observe for signs and symptoms of infection; elevated temperature and WBC. 2. Monitor RR, breath sounds.

(continued)

The Patient With Acute Renal Failure: Intrarenal *(continued)*

NURSING DIAGNOSIS	OUTCOME CRITERIA/ PATIENT GOALS	NURSING ORDERS/INTERVENTIONS
High risk for injury: related to anemia secondary to renal failure.	• Patient will not have anemia.	3. Observe IV insertion sites for signs of inflammation.
		4. Turn, cough, deep-breathe q2h.
		1. Monitor HBF, HCT.
		2. Observe for signs of bleeding; hematest urine and stool.
		3. Observe for symptoms of anemia; increased fatigue, pallor, dyspnea, altered consciousness.
		4. Provide adequate nutrition and rest.
Fluid volume excess: related to ARF, poor filtration, and IV intake.	• Patient will maintain fluid balance.	1. Monitor urine output.
	• Patient's status will be maintained.	2. Record and assess intake and output.
		3. Assess urine for hematuria, specific gravity.
		4. Provide for safety if BUN and creatinine levels are elevated.
		5. Monitor for signs and symptoms of toxic drug accumulation.
		6. Assess lung sounds for crackles and periphery for edema.

The Patient With Acute Renal Failure: Postrenal

NURSING DIAGNOSIS	OUTCOME CRITERIA/ PATIENT GOALS	NURSING ORDERS/INTERVENTIONS
Altered urinary elimination: related to obstruction secondary to cancer of prostate, urethral obstruction.	• Patient will be able to maintain urinary elimination.	1. Observe voiding pattern.
		2. Maintain patency of urinary catheters.
		3. Palpate bladder for retention, catheterize if necessary per physician's order.
		4. Take measures to prevent calculi (ie, change position q2h, administer urine-acidifying juices).
		5. Inspect urine for hematuria and stones.
		6. Provide for privacy during procedures.
	• Patient will maintain fluid and electrolyte balance.	1. Maintain accurate intake and output record.
		2. Replace sodium, potassium, and chloride losses.
		3. Weigh patient daily.
		4. Encourage fluids per physician's order.

(*continued*)

The Patient With Acute Renal Failure: Postrenal (continued)

NURSING DIAGNOSIS	OUTCOME CRITERIA/ PATIENT GOALS	NURSING ORDERS/INTERVENTIONS
High risk for altered comfort: related to ineffective urinary elimination, full bladder.	• Patient will be able to maintain comfort during urinary elimination.	1. Monitor for favorable or adverse responses to treatment regimen.
		2. Administer pain medication per physician's order.
		3. Instruct in nonpharmacologic means of pain relief (ie, relaxation techniques).
		4. Allow patient time and privacy during urination.

The Patient With Congestive Heart Failure and Prerenal Azotemia

NURSING DIAGNOSIS	OUTCOME CRITERIA/ PATIENT GOALS	NURSING ORDERS/INTERVENTIONS
Self-care deficit: feeding, bathing, hygiene and ambulation related to weakness and fatigue secondary to congestive heart failure.	• Patient will show increased independence in carrying out hygiene activities. • Patient will have increased endurance in completing self-care activities.	1. Observe functional level every shift and report any changes. 2. Encourage patient to verbalize concerns about self-care deficits. 3. Monitor completion of bathing and hygiene activities daily. 4. Provide assistance with ambulation as needed. 5. Instruct on bathing techniques that conserve energy. 6. Assist with feeding. 7. Apply lotion to dry, flaky skin areas.
Altered tissue perfusion: related to volume depletion secondary to prerenal azotemia.	• Maintain fluid and electrolyte balance. • Maintain serum sodium within normal limits.	1. Observe voiding pattern. 2. Hydrate per physician's order. 3. Monitor BP, pulse, respirations, and temperature q2h and then q4h.

(continued)

The Patient With Congestive Heart Failure and Prerenal Azotemia *(continued)*

NURSING DIAGNOSIS	OUTCOME CRITERIA/ PATIENT GOALS	NURSING ORDERS/INTERVENTIONS
		4. Maintain intake and output record.
		5. Observe character of urine.
		6. Monitor laboratory reports.
		7. Instruct regarding sodium-restricted diet.
		8. Assist with ambulation when ordered.
		9. Weigh patient daily.
		10. Check skin turgor q4h.
Altered nutrition: less than body requirements: related to loss of appetite and fatigue secondary to congestive heart failure and prerenal azotemia.	• Adequate dietary intake will be promoted.	1. Weigh patient daily.
	• Patient will adhere to 1,200-calorie, 2-g sodium diet.	2. Assist with all meals and snacks.
	• Patient will demonstrate knowledge about need for adequate food and fluid intake.	3. Arrange in a comfortable sitting position.
		4. Remove all noxious stimuli.
		5. Arrange for family member to be present at meal times.

- Patient's energy levels will be maintained.

6. Instruct on rationale for six-meal-a-day diet plan and adequate fluid intake.

7. Arrange for dietitian also to instruct on prescribed diet.

8. Provide for frequent rest before each meal period.

9. Perform range of motion exercises q2h.

The Patient With Cerebral Aneurysm or AVM

NURSING DIAGNOSIS	OUTCOME CRITERIA/ PATIENT GOALS	NURSING ORDERS/INTERVENTIONS
Altered tissue perfusion: related to interruption in cerebral blood flow or increased intracranial pressure.	• Patient will maintain cerebral perfusion pressure of at least 50 mm Hg. • Patient will maintain ICP less than 15 mm Hg. • LOC will not deteriorate below that of baseline.	1. Report cerebral perfusion pressure less than 50 mm Hg. 2. Report ICP rises over 15 mm Hg. 3. Report decrease in Glasgow Coma Scale. 4. Keep head of bed elevated 30° with no neck flexion or hip flexion greater than 90° and no severe head rotation. 5. Minimize frequency and duration of suctioning if it is necessary. Hyperventilate and hyperoxygenate before suctioning, and limit procedure to 10 seconds at a time. 6. Base nursing care activities on ICP. Allow ICP to drop between activities.

7. Coordinate activities with other departments to avoid ICP elevation (eg, x-rays, therapies, etc.), allowing adequate rest periods.

8. Report changes in patient's condition before a critical change in vital signs may alter cerebral perfusion.

9. Provide sedation or analgesia as ordered.

10. Tell patient what is about to be done to him or her before the activity (the brain stem may be intact even though the patient appears nonresponsive).

11. Avoid conversations over the patient's bed that you would not have if he or she were fully awake.

12. Use restraints only when absolutely necessary, because fighting restraints will raise intrathoracic and intraabdominal pressure, thus impeding venous outflow from the head.

13. Allow only passive ROM exercises when ICP is labile.

(continued)

The Patient With Cerebral Aneurysm or AVM *(continued)*

NURSING DIAGNOSIS	OUTCOME CRITERIA/ PATIENT GOALS	NURSING ORDERS/INTERVENTIONS
		14. Calculate CPP if an ICP monitor and an arterial line are in place (CPP = mean systemic arterial pressure minus ICP).
		15. Minimize activity preoperatively, providing a quiet environment.
High risk for sensory–perceptual alteration: related to altered LOC, disorientation, impaired communication skills, restricted and/ or unfamiliar environment.	• Patient will interpret environmental stimuli appropriately.	1. Provide frequent orientation; clock, calendar etc.
		2. Explain unfamiliar machinery, noises, and role of people in patient's environment.
		3. Converse with unconscious patient as if he or she were awake.
		4. Label bedside with patient's perceptual deficit so all caregivers are aware (eg, "patient cannot speak").
		5. Allow for adequate sleep and rest. Alter lighting and reduce auditory stimuli to promote normal circadian sleep patterns.

6. Provide alternate communication method if unable to verbalize (eg, alphabet chart).

7. Apply coma stimulation techniques to awaken patient from coma.

8. Encourage family visits and verbalization to patient and suggest they bring in personal items, such as pictures, to help reorient patient.

High risk for pain: related to meningeal signs (stiff neck, headache, photophobia) from subarachnoid hemorrhage.

• Patient will rate discomfort less than 4 on a scale of 1–10 (1 being minimal pain and 10 being excruciating).

1. Teach patient to use a pain rating scale before administration of analgesics and 30 min after administration.

2. Position to prevent neck flexion or hip flexion over 90°.

3. Keep room dark to minimize photophobia.

4. Keep environment quiet.

5. Administer analgesics around the clock, as ordered, to prevent pain from getting out of control.

(continued)

The Patient With Cerebral Aneurysm or AVM (continued)

NURSING DIAGNOSIS	OUTCOME CRITERIA/ PATIENT GOALS	NURSING ORDERS/INTERVENTIONS
High risk for altered fluid volume excess related to neuro/hormonal dysfunction of hypervolemia used to treat vasospasm or deficit related to fluid restriction and use of osmotics to control ICP.	• Patient will maintain adequate hydration.	1. Record intake and output, vital signs, and hemodynamic parameters at least q4h.
		2. Report signs of fluid overload: tachypnea, tachycardia, neck vein distention, edema, gallop rhythm.
		3. Report signs of fluid volume deficit: hypotension, oliguria, dry mucous membranes, poor skin turgor, complaints of thirst.
		4. Auscultate and record breath sounds frequently.
		5. Calculate fluid balance at least q24h.
		6. Use an IV pump for accurate administration of fluids.
		7. Report signs of increased ICP or change in LOC.
		8. Monitor serum electrolyte values.

The Patient With Increased Intracranial Pressure

NURSING DIAGNOSIS	OUTCOME CRITERIA/ PATIENT GOALS	NURSING ORDERS/INTERVENTIONS
Altered tissue perfusion: related to decreased space for cerebral perfusion, cerebral tissue edema, decreased perfusion systemically, or absent cerebral perfusion due to embolus or cerebral vascular flow interruption.	• The patient's level of consciousness will be improved or maintained.	1. Accurately measure ICP and follow measurements continuously.
		2. Document ICP measurement q1h and as changes occur.
		3. Evaluate pattern of ICP monitoring to verify accuracy of the readings.
		4. Elevate head of bed 15°–30° at all times.
		5. Avoid flexion of the neck and head turning.
		6. Promote venous drainage of skull with alignment of the head.
		7. Use a consistent neurologic assessment system, such as the Glasgow Coma Scale. There must be consistency between nurses for an accurate trend of assessment data.

(continued)

The Patient With Increased Intracranial Pressure (continued)

NURSING DIAGNOSIS	OUTCOME CRITERIA/ PATIENT GOALS	NURSING ORDERS / INTERVENTIONS
		8. Evaluate the following q1h and prn: Level of consciousness Pupil size Pupil reaction to light (briskness and size) Equality of pupils Movement of extremities Least stimulus to get reaction from the patient Appropriateness of patient's response to environment or stimuli Presence or absence of reflexes All involuntary motion such as seizures, twitching or asymmetry of motor function Blood pressure Heart rate and rhythm Respiratory rate and rhythm Hemodynamic parameters (PAP, PAd, PCWP, CVP, CO, CI) as available by invasive lines

9. Calculate the CPP q1h and prn (CPP = MAP − ICP)

10. Report changes in assessment or CPP <70 or >90 mm Hg to physician.

11. Avoid increases in intrathoracic pressure: avoid the use of PEEP on mechanical ventilators; avoid hip flexion; avoid coughing, vomiting, or Valsalva maneuvers.

12. If ventilation is controlled with mechanical ventilator, keep PCO_2 low (18–25) to prevent cerebral vasodilatation.

13. Control environment to decrease stimulation, limit contact with patient to necessary procedures.

14. Administer corticosteroids, as ordered.

15. Administer diuretics that decrease tissue volume (such as mannitol), as ordered.

(continued)

The Patient With Increased Intracranial Pressure *(continued)*

NURSING DIAGNOSIS	OUTCOME CRITERIA/ PATIENT GOALS	NURSING ORDERS/INTERVENTIONS
		16. Maintain an accurate input and output, q8h.
		17. Limit fluid intake as much as possible.
		18. Anticipate dehydration, monitor urine and serum Na, osmolality.
		19. Maintain normal temperature, prevent shivering.
		20. Provide sedation or sedation and paralysis, as ordered, with barbiturates or Pavulon.
		21. Provide hyperventilation before removal from mechanical ventilator for suctioning.
Fluid volume deficit: related to diabetes insipidus (DI), potential diuretic therapy, high metabolic needs, diaphoresis, renal failure.	• Minimal intake and adequate output will be maintained.	1. Monitor the trends in serum and urine Na, osmolality, and creatinine levels.
		2. Keep accurate input and output q8h.
		3. Do not move patient to weigh (increased stimuli) unless absolutely necessary.

4. Give medications (IVPB antibiotics) in minimal volumes.

5. Assess for DI: high urine output with low specific gravity.

6. Replace electrolytes with supplemental therapy, as ordered.

7. If DI present give Pitressin and DDAVP, as ordered.

8. Monitor CVP and hemodynamic data, as available.

Ineffective breathing pattern: related to subdued level of consciousness, brain tissue injury near medulla or pons, inability to maintain adequate airway, lack of control over respiratory muscles, severe hypoventilation, or pulmonary complications.

• Patent airway will be maintained.

1. Assess ability to maintain patent airway.

2. Assess reflexes necessary for adequate breathing: cough, gag, and swallow.

3. Assess respirations for rate, depth, regularity, and chest expansion.

4. Assess breath sounds for the movement of air to all lung fields.

5. Maintain an elevated head of bed.

6. Assess ABGs for evidence of adequate gas exchange, qd and prn.

7. If mechanical ventilation is needed, maintain hyperventilation.

(continued)

The Patient With Increased Intracranial Pressure *(continued)*

NURSING DIAGNOSIS	OUTCOME CRITERIA/ PATIENT GOALS	NURSING ORDERS/INTERVENTIONS
		8. Be aware of impact of depressant or sedative drugs on the respiratory drive.
		9. Suction, as needed, providing hyperventilation before the procedure.
		10. Monitor heart rate and rhythm.
		11. Follow results of daily chest x-ray reports.
		12. Monitor oxygenation with pulse oximetry.
High risk for altered body temperature: related to brain tissue injury or infection.	• Body temperature will stay within normal limits.	1. Check core temperature frequently.
		2. Prevent shivering by lowering an elevated temperature slowly.
		3. Use cooling blanket, as ordered.
		4. Administer antipyretics, such as Tylenol, as ordered.
		5. Administer antibiotics, as ordered.
		6. Control the environmental temperature.

High risk for infection: related to invasive lines, decreased level of consciousness and immobility.

- Nosocomial infection will not occur.

7. Maintain aseptic technique with all procedures.

1. Use strict sterile technique during insertion of ICP monitoring device, and maintenance of external ventricular drainage system.

2. Perform sterile dressing changes at ICP monitoring device site, qd.

3. Assess for symptoms of CNS infection: changes in LOC; increased WBC; elevated temperature; nuchal rigidity; photophobia; positive Kernig's sign.

4. Obtain CSF cultures, as ordered.

5. Administer antibiotics, as ordered.

6. Monitor and record the presence of leaking CSF from nose, ears, or ICP monitoring device site.

(continued)

The Patient With Increased Intracranial Pressure *(continued)*

NURSING DIAGNOSIS	OUTCOME CRITERIA/ PATIENT GOALS	NURSING ORDERS/INTERVENTIONS
High risk for injury: related to decreased level of consciousness, agitation, restlessness, or involuntary motion such as seizure activity.	• Patient will be free from injury.	1. Evaluate the patient's potential risk for injury, q8h and prn.
		2. If restless, pad side rails, keep both side rails up, keep bed in low position and restrain patient with soft wrist restraints or vest/jacket restraint, as needed.
		3. If subdued level of consciousness, turn q2h, position in anatomically functional positions, use soft wrist restraints, use device to decrease the stiffness of the mattress; keep side rails up and the bed in low position.
		4. Perform passive ROM exercises, if not contraindicated by increased ICP.
		5. Maintain bronchial hygiene.
		6. Position to prevent aspirations.
		7. Use antiembolism stockings.
		8. Use high-top tennis shoes to prevent footdrop.

9. Assess integrity of skin q8h.

10. Keep skin clean, dry, free of harsh soaps or chemicals.

11. Promote mobility and place patient in the chair, as soon as medically cleared for increased activities.

High risk for altered nutrition: related to decreased level of consciousness, mechanical ventilation, or increased metabolic needs.

• Adequate nutrition will be maintained.

1. Maintain NPO status until full assessment is complete.

2. Evaluate cough, gag, and swallow reflexes.

3. Auscultate abdomen for bowel sounds q8h.

4. If patient able to chew and swallow, feed patient a balanced diet including foods of the patient's choice.

5. If unable to masticate and swallow, place thin, soft-walled feeding tube, as ordered.

(continued)

The Patient With Increased Intracranial Pressure (continued)

NURSING DIAGNOSIS	OUTCOME CRITERIA/ PATIENT GOALS	NURSING ORDERS/INTERVENTIONS
		6. Verify feeding tube placement with radiography initially, and q8h with auscultation for injected air, aspiration of contents with syringe, or injection of water.
		7. Initiate tube feedings with small amounts and lower concentration. Increase amount and strength, as tolerated and as ordered.
		8. Stop any tube feeding if residual in stomach is large or regurgitation occurs.
		9. Maintain an elevated head of the bed during all tube feedings.
		10. Limit diarrhea with antidiarrheal agents.
		11. Give calories and free water, either by mouth or feeding tube.
		12. Weigh qd, when ICP has stabilized.
		13. Monitor fluid and electrolyte balance, qd and prn.

The Patient With a Stroke

NURSING DIAGNOSIS

Altered thought process: related to left hemispheric stroke manifested by possible speech involvement, right hemiplegia, dysphasia (expressive or receptive); slow, cautious disorganized behavior, right visual field cut, high level of frustration.

OUTCOME CRITERIA/ PATIENT GOALS

- Patient will be able to cope with the deficit, as demonstrated by interacting with others without evidence of prolonged or frequent frustration.

NURSING ORDERS/INTERVENTIONS

1. Initiate neurologic rehabilitation, including occupational therapy, physical therapy, speech therapy, cognitive therapy, and others as indicated.

2. Encourage use of facilitative equipment to improve speech or communication (eg, writing board, picture board, alphabet board).

3. Speak slowly to patient and allow adequate time for response; avoid speaking to patient as if a child.

4. Help patient establish a daily routine schedule to follow to help organize behavior.

5. Provide orientation to environment through use of clock, calendar, pictures, and verbalization.

6. Organize care to occur within visual field on left, when possible.

(continued)

The Patient With a Stroke (continued)

NURSING DIAGNOSIS	OUTCOME CRITERIA/PATIENT GOALS	NURSING ORDERS/INTERVENTIONS
Altered thought process: related to right hemispheric stroke manifested by possible left hemiplegia, spatial perceptual deficits, memory deficits, emotional lability, left hemianopsia, apraxia, or poor judgment.	• Patient will be able to cope with the deficit, as demonstrated by use of pencil and paper to augment memory, compensation for unilateral neglect, and absence of frequent emotional outbursts.	1. Participate in neurologic rehabilitation consultation. 2. Promote awareness of body and environment on the affected side. 3. Divide tasks into simple steps; elicit return demonstration of skills. 4. Use nonverbal clues to enhance patient understanding. 5. Use slow minimal movements and avoid clutter around the patient. 6. Provide emotional support to patient/family. Allow ventilation. Explain to family the reason for patient's emotional lability. 7. Position patient in bed to prevent falls. Consider posey restraints and side rails.

8. Reorient patient to environment frequently through use of clock, calendar, radio, etc.

9. Encourage use of notebook to write down things patient needs to remember, and to carry the notebook with him or her.

10. Use brief periods of teaching, because attention span is limited, and divide tasks into multiple simple steps.

11. Assure that medications will be given under supervision at home so patient does not forget to take them and takes the correct dose.

High risk for altered tissue perfusion: related to interruption in cerebral blood flow, cerebral hemorrhaging, increased ICP.

• Patient will maintain cerebral perfusion pressure of at least 60 mm Hg and ICP of less than 20 mm Hg.

1. Enhance venous outflow from the head by keeping head of bed elevated without neck flexion or severe head rotation.

2. Avoid or minimize frequency and duration of nursing care which may increase intraabdominal or intrathoracic pressure (eg, suctioning).

(continued)

The Patient With a Stroke *(continued)*

NURSING DIAGNOSIS	OUTCOME CRITERIA/ PATIENT GOALS	NURSING ORDERS/INTERVENTIONS
		3. Check tape around endotracheal tube or tracheostomy to ensure ties are not tight enough to impede cerebral blood flow.
		4. Maintain normothermia.
		5. Avoid use of restraints if possible, because the ICP will increase and CPP will decrease if patient fights against them.
		6. Report increased systolic BP, widening pulse pressure, bradycardia, headache, vomiting, and papilledema, all of which might indicate herniation.
		7. Prevent constipation. Record all bowel movements.
		8. Document neurologic status using Glasgow Coma Scale and compare with baseline.
		9. Report changes in level of consciousness.

High risk for injury: related to seizure activity, altered thought processes, immobility, impaired self-protective mechanisms, motor weakness, impulsiveness, decreased level of responsiveness, or dysphagia/aspiration.

- Level of consciousness will be maintained or improved.
- Patient will be free from physical injury.

1. Use seizure precautions: side rails up and padded, bed in low position, tongue blade or airway available, oxygen and suction at bedside.

2. Accurately observe and record seizure.

3. Assist unsteady or ataxic patient to ambulate.

4. Teach self-protective actions (eg, teach patient to scan total environment with head to make up for visual field cut on one side).

5. Assure adequate swallow, gag, and cough reflexes before offering oral fluids and food.

6. Teach family to assess home environment for hazards (eg, throw rugs, stairs without railings, bathroom without grab bars, etc.).

7. Teach family what to do if patient seizes after discharge from the hospital.

(continued)

The Patient With a Stroke (continued)

NURSING DIAGNOSIS	OUTCOME CRITERIA/ PATIENT GOALS	NURSING ORDERS/INTERVENTIONS
High risk for altered nutrition, less than body requirements: related to muscle weakness during swallowing, confusion, depression, critical illness, or inability to feed self.	• Patient will take in adequate calories to meet body's metabolic demands, as measured by calorie count and calculation of metabolic requirements.	1. Document calorie count daily. 2. Initiate dietary consultation. 3. Administer tube feedings, total parenteral nutrition, or assist with oral feeding based on patient's condition. 4. Assess serum albumin, total protein, and WBC. 5. Maintain daily weight record.
High risk for impaired physical mobility: related to hemiparesis, hemiplegia, contractures, foot drop, muscle atrophy, pain, altered level of consciousness, or fatigue.	• Patient will be free of preventable complications of immobility such as atelectasis, pressure sores, and deep vein thrombosis.	1. Initiate rehabilitation consultation. 2. Perform passive/active ROM tid and record. 3. Provide space boots or high-top tennis shoes. 4. Apply splints if needed, as directed by physical therapy. 5. Mobilize patient to chair as soon as possible. 6. Position patient correctly with pillows while in bed.

7. Turn patient q2h.

8. Provide egg-crate mattress, sheep skin, or consider kinetic bed as indicated.

9. Provide heel and elbow protectors.

10. Ensure adequate nutrition.

11. Teach patient to use spirometry or to cough/deep breathe frequently, or suction as needed to keep lungs clear.

12. Assess lower extremities frequently for redness, tenderness, warmth, or pain.

13. Apply elastic stockings or pneumatic stockings while immobile.

The Patient With Acute Pancreatitis

NURSING DIAGNOSIS

Fluid volume deficit: related to fluid se-questration due to activated pancreatic en-zymes in peritoneum; vomiting; prolonged NG suction; potential hemorrhage into the pancreas.

OUTCOME CRITERIA/ PATIENT GOALS

• Patient will remain hemodynamically stable.

NURSING ORDERS / INTERVENTIONS

1. Monitor vital signs and urine output q1h and prn; skin turgor capillary refill, peripheral pulses, q4h and prn.

2. Monitor hemodynamic values if pul-monary artery catheter is placed; PCWP, CVP, SVR, cardiac output, and cardiac index.

3. Maintain patent IV line; central line preferred.

4. Administer fluid replacements (eg, colloids, crystalloids, blood or blood products) and monitor patient re-sponse.

5. Maintain and evaluate intake and output records.

6. Weigh patient daily on same scale at same time.

7. Monitor of signs and symptoms of hemorrhage: hematocrit and hemoglobin q2h; Cullen or Turner's sign.

8. Measure abdominal girth q4h.

9. Monitor electrolytes, CBC, and coagulation factors; replace electrolytes as prescribed.

10. Monitor renal function studies (eg, BUN, creatinine, urinary Na, osmolality).

11. Place patient on bed rest.

12. Maintain NPO status.

Pain: related to interruption of blood supply to the pancreas; edema and distention of the pancreas; peritoneal irritation from activated pancreatic exocrine enzymes.

- Patient reports pain is within tolerable limits.

1. Perform a pain assessment noting onset, duration, intensity, and location.

2. Instruct patient on use of a 0–10 pain rating scale.

3. Assess patient anxiety.

4. Administer non-opiate analgesic; schedule pain medication regularly to prevent severe pain episodes.

4. Keep activities at a minimum. Maintain bed rest restriction. Position patient to optimize comfort.

(continued)

The Patient With Acute Pancreatitis (*continued*)

NURSING DIAGNOSIS	OUTCOME CRITERIA/ PATIENT GOALS	NURSING ORDERS/INTERVENTIONS
		5. Provide comfort measures; mouth care, positioning; control fever.
Altered nutrition, less than body requirements: related to prolonged NPO status; nausea and vomiting; depressed appetite; impaired nutrient metabolism due to pancreatic injury and altered production of digestive enzymes.	• Nutritional needs of patient will be adequately met.	1. Assess nutritional status through clinical exam and laboratory analysis.
		2. Calculate caloric needs and compare to actual intake.
		3. Administer TPN as ordered. Avoid lipid therapy.
		4. Prevent complications by attention to aseptic technique in the handling and administration of TPN and catheter care.
		5. Monitor for signs and symptoms of infection.
		6. Monitor glucose, albumin, and electrolytes to detect complications of therapy.
		7. Assess acid–base balance with ABGs.

Impaired gas exchange: related to atelectasis; pleural effusions; ARDS; fluid overload during fluid administration; pulmonary emboli; splinting from pain.

- Patient will have adequate breathing pattern and gas exchange.

1. Monitor pulmonary status closely. Auscultate breath sounds q2–4h and prn; monitor respiratory rate, chest excursion and symmetry; assess for signs of respiratory distress.

2. Administer vigorous pulmonary hygiene; coughing and deep breathing; humidification therapy.

3. Note secretions for amount, color, consistency, and odor.

4. Administer oxygen as prescribed.

5. Monitor with oximetry for SaO_2.

6. Administer analgesia to prevent splinting due to pain.

7. Reposition patient frequently to maximize ventilation and perfusion and to prevent pooling of secretions.

8. Assist with paracentesis as ordered when ascites compromises respiratory status.

The Patient in Adrenal Crisis

NURSING DIAGNOSIS

Fluid volume deficit: related to loss of sodium and water associated with adrenal insufficiency.

OUTCOME CRITERIA / PATIENT GOALS

- Fluid volume and electrolytes will return to normal.

NURSING ORDERS / INTERVENTIONS

1. Administer intravenous fluids (usually D5%/NS) with electrolyte replacements, as ordered. Initial volume replacement may be rapid to restore intravascular volume.

2. Administer scheduled doses of intravenous hydrocortisone, as ordered.

3. Monitor serum electrolyte levels; assess for signs and symptoms of hyponatremia and hyperkalemia.

4. Assess cardiovascular function: BP, HR, rhythm (ie, dysthrythmias, bradycardia).

5. Monitor urinary specific gravity q4h.

6. Assess neuromuscular status; weakness, twitching, hyperreflexia, paresthesia.

Decreased cardiac output: related to hypovolemic vascular shock associated with adrenal insufficiency.

• Hemodynamic stability will be maintained.

7. Conserve energy stores initially by providing rest periods, and assist with ADLs.

1. Assess cardiac workload q15min: BP, orthostatic hypotension, central venous pressure, skin color and temperature, capillary refills, and presence of subjective symptoms.

2. Monitor urinary output q1h.

3. Administer vasoconstrictive agents, as ordered.

The Patient With Diabetic Ketoacidosis

NURSING DIAGNOSIS	OUTCOME CRITERIA/ PATIENT GOALS	NURSING ORDERS/INTERVENTIONS
Fluid volume deficit: related to hyperglycemia secondary to diabetes ketoacidosis (DKA).	• Restore fluid and electrolyte balance.	1. Administer intravenous fluids, insulin, and, as needed, electrolyte replacements, per physician's order.
		2. Monitor laboratory reports (ie, Hct, Hgb, sodium, chloride, magnesium, BUN, creatinine, phosphate, CO_2, HCO_3^-, and pH).
		3. Monitor hydration q1/2h to q1h initially: intake and output, urine specific gravity, skin moisture, and turgor.
		4. Monitor blood pressure, temperature, and pulse q1h initially, then q4h.
		5. Monitor ECG strips for indications of electrolyte changes q1h.
	• Slowly bring serum glucose within normal limits.	6. Monitor blood glucose q1/2h until stable, also urine ketones.

7. Observe for signs of electrolyte and acid–base imbalance (ie, "fruity" odor of breath, cherry red color of skin and mucous membranes, tetany, carpopedal spasm, neuromuscular irritability, and seizures).

8. Evaluate mental status q1h until crises subside, and q4h thereafter.

- Resolution of nausea and vomiting, abdominal pain, tenderness, and rigidity.

1. Provide care measures for nasogastric intubation.

2. Maintain gastric decompression.

3. Monitor bowel sounds q2h.

4. Assist with oral hygiene q2h.

5. Withhold food and fluids, per physician's order.

6. Provide ice chips, per physician's order. Fluid restriction as ordered.

7. Record color, amount, and frequency of vomiting.

- Promote normal nutrition as appetite improves and symptoms decrease.

1. Provide calm atmosphere during meals.

2. Involve patient in diet plan.

(continued)

The Patient With Diabetic Ketoacidosis (continued)

NURSING DIAGNOSIS	OUTCOME CRITERIA/ PATIENT GOALS	NURSING ORDERS/INTERVENTIONS
		3. Identify factors (eg, depression, acid-base imbalance) that may contribute to loss of appetite.
		4. Minimize unpleasant sights and odors in immediate environment.
High risk for impaired gas exchange: related to pneumonia, DKA Kussmal respirations.	• Resolve infectious process.	1. Identify factors contributing to decreased resistance to infection.
		2. Monitor temperature q4h.
		3. Observe for signs and symptoms of infection (eg, fatigue, elevated WBC, elevated temperature).
		4. Promote rest.
	• Promote natural gas exchanges and breathing pattern.	1. Monitor results of chest film.
		2. Auscultate lungs q1h until stable, then q4h.
		3. Elevate head of bed to facilitate breathing comfort.
		4. Assess respiratory rate and depth q4h.
		5. Perform pulmonary toilet, per physician's order.

Knowledge deficit: related to inability to manage episode of diabetic crisis.

- Patient can explain physiological stressors that may precipitate diabetic ketoacidosis.

1. Assess patient's knowledge of precipitating factors and sick day guidelines.

2. Instruct on events that could precipitate diabetic ketoacidosis (eg, infection, injury, or emotional stress).

- Patient and family can state 5 sick day guidelines.

3. Instruct or review sick day guidelines concerning

    administering insulin;

    food and fluid intake;

    testing blood or urine for glucose and urine for ketones;

    notifying health provider to inform and receive further direction;

    emergency resources.

- Patient and family can identify symptoms requiring medical/nursing intervention.

4. Instruct patient and family in signs and symptoms of diabetic emergencies.

5. Instruct on importance of having sufficient insulin on hand.

6. Provide names and telephone numbers of resource persons to contact if problems arise.

7. Instruct patient to wear medical identification bracelet.

The Patient With Myxedema Coma

NURSING DIAGNOSIS	OUTCOME CRITERIA/ PATIENT GOALS	NURSING ORDERS/INTERVENTIONS
Altered tissue perfusion, cerebral: related to hypothyroidism.	• Patient will return to usual wakeful state.	1. Implement seizure precautions. 2. Closely monitor patient's neurological status for changes in LOC. 3. Monitor patient's ability to protect airway, effectively cough and gag. 4. Administer thyroid replacement therapy (thyroxine), and glucocorticoids, as ordered.
Hypothermia: related to decreased metabolic state.	• Body temperature will return to patient's norm.	1. Assess temperature q1h. 2. Implement measures to raise body temperature; gradual warming is recommended.

High risk for injury: related to decreased level of consciousness and hypothyroid state.	• Patient will be injury and infection free.	1. Prevent infection. Monitor clinical signs and symptoms. A normothermic patient may indicate an infectious process.
		2. Provide skin and other supportive care required for an immobile patient.
Cardiac output: related to decreased inotropic state.	• Hemodynamic stability will be maintained.	1. Administer fluid therapy that is dependent on patient's clinical status.
		2. Monitor therapy to prevent fluid overload.
		3. Assess PB, HR, T, and rhythm q15min until stable.

The Patient With AIDS

NURSING DIAGNOSIS	OUTCOME CRITERIA/ PATIENT GOALS	NURSING ORDERS/INTERVENTIONS
High risk for infection: related to HIV immunodeficiency and malnutrition.	• Patient will be free from nosocomial infections.	1. Use universal precautions.
		2. Assess baseline immunologic studies: T cell count, WBC, differential.
		3. Stress proper handwashing techniques by all caregivers.
		4. Monitor visitors/caregivers to protect compromised host.
		5. Monitor for signs and symptoms of sepsis: fever, hypotension, positive blood cultures.
		6. Assist patient and family in learning about preventing infection.
High risk for impaired gas exchange: related to alveolar–capillary membrane changes with PCP infection.	• Patient will maintain adequate oxygenation.	1. Monitor for signs and symptoms of respiratory compromise: tachypnea, cyanosis, changes in mentation, fatigue.
		2. Review pertinent laboratory data: CBC, chest radiograph, ABG.

3. Assess activity tolerance.

4. Administer oxygen.

5. Monitor therapeutic and adverse effects of antibiotic therapy.

6. Monitor oxygen saturation with oximetry.

High risk for fluid volume deficit: related to diarrhea, dysphagia.

• Patient will maintain fluid and electrolyte balance.

1. Assess risk factors: fever, diarrhea, dysphagia.

2. Monitor weight and intake and output.

3. Assess vital sign changes: hypotension, tachycardia, fever.

4. Encourage increased oral intake of fluids.

5. Provide supplemental fluids, as ordered: IV, tube feeding.

6. Administer medications, as ordered (antidiarrheals, antipyretics).

7. Assess lab data, as ordered.

High risk for altered thought processes: related to HIV or opportunistic infection of CNS.

• Patient will maintain or improve level of consciousness.

1. Assess neurologic status q4h.

2. Assess for changes in behavior, slowing and slurring of speech.

3. Maintain safe environment.

(continued)

The Patient With AIDS (continued)

NURSING DIAGNOSIS	OUTCOME CRITERIA/ PATIENT GOALS	NURSING ORDERS/ INTERVENTIONS
High risk for knowledge deficit: related to illness and impact on patient's future.	• Patient will verbalize understanding of AIDS and treatment.	1. Initiate nurse–patient relationship to encourage learning.
		2. Include family in teaching.
		3. Provide discharge teaching that emphasizes avoidance of exposure to infection, safe sex practices, diet, and maintaining high level of wellness.
		4. Assist patient in identifying community support groups and resources available.
High risk for anxiety: related to critical illness, fear of death.	• Patient will begin to identify source of anxiety.	1. Provide environment that encourages open discussion of emotional issues.
		2. Mobilize patient's support system and involve these resources as appropriate.
		3. Allow time for patient to express self.
		4. Identify possible hospital resources for patient and family support.
		5. Encourage open family-to-nurse communications regarding emotional issues.

High risk for infection transmission: related to AIDS.

- Patient will not contaminate health care team, other patients, or family.

6. Validate patient and family knowledge base regarding the critical illness.

7. Involve religious support systems as appropriate.

1. Use universal precautions with every patient.

2. Instruct patient to handwash after handling own secretions.

3. Use extra care with disposal of body secretions, needles.

4. Use "needleless" IV system for IVPB meds, etc.

5. Observe all health team members' technique for universal precautions, and give feedback.

The Patient With Cocaine Toxicity

NURSING DIAGNOSIS	OUTCOME CRITERIA/ PATIENT GOALS	NURSING ORDERS/INTERVENTIONS
High risk for altered cardiac tissue perfusion: related to dysrhythmias and increased myocardial oxygen demand.	• Vital signs will return to or remain within normal limits.	1. Assess vital signs q15min initially and prn. 2. Note changes in blood pressure, heart rate, and rhythm. 3. Maintain bed rest. 4. Auscultate heart sounds q2h and prn. 5. Administer oxygen and medications, as ordered. 6. Monitor pulse oximetry or arterial blood gases, as ordered.
Hyperthermia: related to drug toxicity.	• Normal body temperature will be maintained.	1. Monitor temperature q15min initially and prn. 2. Place patient in cool room. 3. Minimize physical activity. 4. Sponge patient with tepid water. 5. Institute external cooling therapies as ordered (eg, cooling blanket).

High risk for injury: related to seizures, restlessness, and agitation.

- Patient will remain free of physical injury.

1. Monitor for seizure activity.
2. Pad side rails.
3. Place oral airway at bedside.
4. Suction equipment available at bedside.
5. Place bed in lower position, all side rails elevated.
6. Administer anticonvulsants, as ordered.
7. Administer sedation, as ordered.
8. Use soft restraints for agitation (not for seizure control).

Anxiety: related to use of a stimulant fear of the unknown, or fear of legal repercussions.

- Patient will demonstrate effective coping skills.

1. Decrease environmental stimuli.
2. Acknowledge and support effective coping mechanisms used by patient.
3. Identify major support systems or people.
4. Enlist patient's cooperation and allow him or her to participate in care when possible.
5. Explain all procedures in simple terms.

(continued)

The Patient With Cocaine Toxicity (continued)

NURSING DIAGNOSIS	OUTCOME CRITERIA/ PATIENT GOALS	NURSING ORDERS/INTERVENTIONS
Knowledge deficit: related to cocaine abuse.	• Patient will verbalize understanding of the physical manifestations of cocaine abuse.	1. Assess patient's and family's understanding of cocaine toxicity and treatment.
		2. Assess learning ability and readiness to learn.
		3. Provide information about the physical effects of cocaine abuse.
		4. Clarify misconceptions.

APPENDIX
ACLS Guidelines for Non–Life-Threatening Situations

Bradycardia Algorithm

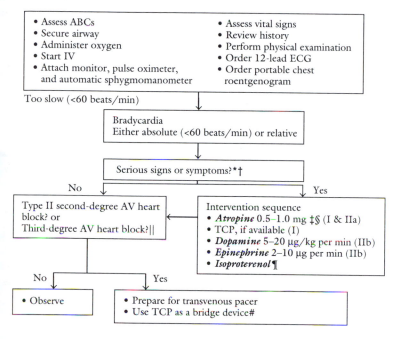

* Serious signs or symptoms must be related to the slow rate.
  Clinical manifestations include:
  symptoms (chest pain, shortness of breath, decreased level of consciousness) and
  signs (low BP, shock, pulmonary congestion, CHF, acute MI).
† Do not delay TCP while awaiting IV access or for *atropine* to take effect if patient is
  symptomatic.
‡ Denervated transplanted hearts will not respond to *atropine*. Go at once to pacing,
  catecholamine infusion, or both.
§ *Atropine* should be given in repeat doses in 3–5 min up to total of 0.04 mg/kg. Consider
  shorter dosing intervals in severe clinical conditions. It has been suggested that atropine
  should be used with caution in atrioventricular (AV) block at the His-Purkinje level (type
  II AV block and new third-degree block with wide QRS complexes) (Class IIb).
‖ Never treat third-degree heart block plus ventricular escape beats with *lidocaine*.
¶ *Isoproterenol* should be used, if at all, with extreme caution. At low doses it is Class IIb
  (possibly helpful); at higher doses it is Class III (harmful).
Verify patient tolerance and mechanical capture. Use analgesia and sedation as needed.

Fig. 5. Bradycardia algorithm (with the patient not in cardiac arrest). (JAMA 268[16]:2221.)

Electrical Cardioversion Algorithm

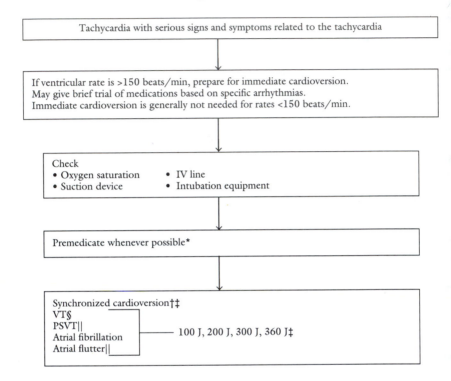

Tachycardia with serious signs and symptoms related to the tachycardia

If ventricular rate is >150 beats/min, prepare for immediate cardioversion.
May give brief trial of medications based on specific arrhythmias.
Immediate cardioversion is generally not needed for rates <150 beats/min.

Check
- Oxygen saturation
- Suction device
- IV line
- Intubation equipment

Premedicate whenever possible*

Synchronized cardioversion†‡
VT§
PSVT‖
Atrial fibrillation
Atrial flutter‖ ———— 100 J, 200 J, 300 J, 360 J‡

* Effective regimens have included a sedative (eg, *diazepam, midazolam, barbiturates, etomidate, ketamine, methohexital*) with or without an analgesic agent (eg, *fentanyl, morphine, meperidine*).
  Many experts recommend anesthesia if service is readily available.
† Note possible need to resynchronize after each cardioversion.
‡ If delays in synchronization occur and clinical conditions are critical, go to immediate unsynchronized shocks.
§ Treat polymorphic VT (irregular form and rate) like VF: 200 J, 200–300 J, 360 J.
‖ PSVT and atrial flutter often respond to lower energy levels (start with 50 J).

Fig. 7. Electrical cardioversion algorithm (with the patient not in cardiac arrest). (JAMA 268[16]:2224.)

Acute Myocardial Infarction (AMI) Algorithm

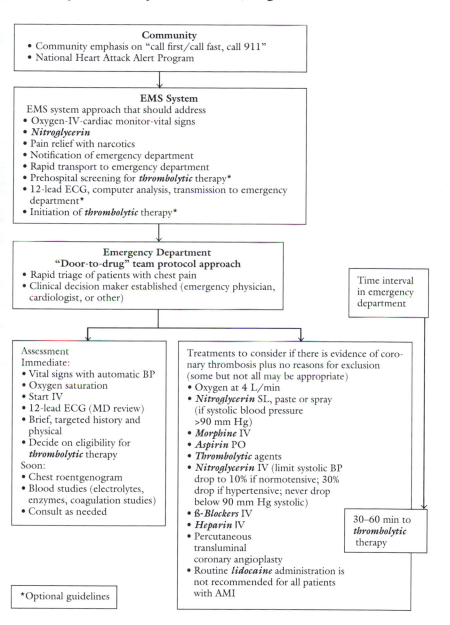

Community
- Community emphasis on "call first/call fast, call 911"
- National Heart Attack Alert Program

EMS System
EMS system approach that should address
- Oxygen-IV-cardiac monitor-vital signs
- *Nitroglycerin*
- Pain relief with narcotics
- Notification of emergency department
- Rapid transport to emergency department
- Prehospital screening for *thrombolytic* therapy*
- 12-lead ECG, computer analysis, transmission to emergency department*
- Initiation of *thrombolytic* therapy*

Emergency Department
"Door-to-drug" team protocol approach
- Rapid triage of patients with chest pain
- Clinical decision maker established (emergency physician, cardiologist, or other)

Time interval in emergency department

Assessment
Immediate:
- Vital signs with automatic BP
- Oxygen saturation
- Start IV
- 12-lead ECG (MD review)
- Brief, targeted history and physical
- Decide on eligibility for *thrombolytic* therapy
Soon:
- Chest roentgenogram
- Blood studies (electrolytes, enzymes, coagulation studies)
- Consult as needed

Treatments to consider if there is evidence of coronary thrombosis plus no reasons for exclusion (some but not all may be appropriate)
- Oxygen at 4 L/min
- *Nitroglycerin* SL, paste or spray (if systolic blood pressure >90 mm Hg)
- *Morphine* IV
- *Aspirin* PO
- *Thrombolytic* agents
- *Nitroglycerin* IV (limit systolic BP drop to 10% if normotensive; 30% drop if hypertensive; never drop below 90 mm Hg systolic)
- ß-*Blockers* IV
- *Heparin* IV
- Percutaneous transluminal coronary angioplasty
- Routine *lidocaine* administration is not recommended for all patients with AMI

30–60 min to *thrombolytic* therapy

*Optional guidelines

Fig. 9. Acute myocardial infarction (AMI) algorithm. Recommendations for early treatment of patients with chest pain and possible AMI. (JAMA 268[16]:2230.)

Algorithm for Hypotension, Shock, and Acute Pulmonary Edema

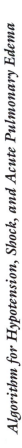
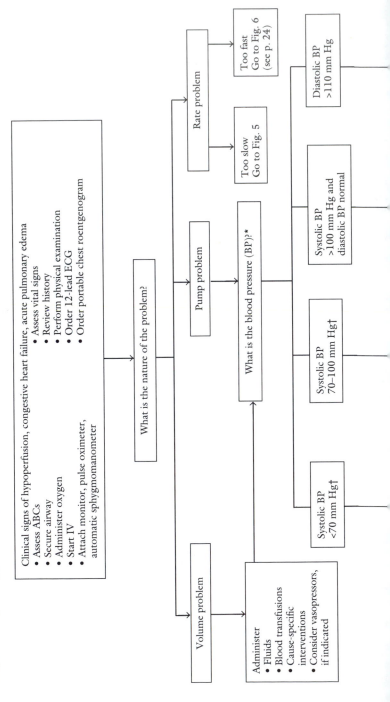

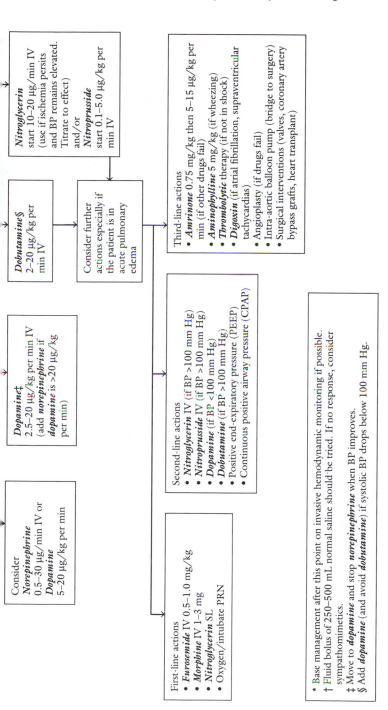

First-line actions
- **Furosemide** IV 0.5–1.0 mg/kg
- **Morphine** IV 1–3 mg
- **Nitroglycerin** SL
- Oxygen/intubate PRN

Second-line actions
- **Nitroglycerin** IV (if BP >100 mm Hg)
- **Nitroprusside** IV (if BP >100 mm Hg)
- **Dopamine** (if BP <100 mm Hg)
- **Dobutamine** (if BP >100 mm Hg)
- Positive end-expiratory pressure (PEEP)
- Continuous positive airway pressure (CPAP)

Third-line actions
- **Amrinone** 0.75 mg/kg then 5–15 μg/kg per min (if other drugs fail)
- **Aminophylline** 5 mg/kg (if wheezing)
- **Thrombolytic** therapy (if not in shock)
- **Digoxin** (if atrial fibrillation, supraventricular tachycardias)
- Angioplasty (if drugs fail)
- Intra-aortic balloon pump (bridge to surgery)
- Surgical interventions (valves, coronary artery bypass grafts, heart transplant)

Consider
Norepinephrine 0.5–30 μg/min IV or *Dopamine* 5–20 μg/kg per min

Dopamine†
2.5–20 μg/kg per min IV (add *norepinephrine* if *dopamine* is >20 μg/kg per min)

Dobutamine§
2–20 μg/kg per min IV

Consider further actions especially if the patient is in acute pulmonary edema

Nitroglycerin
start 10–20 μg/min IV (use if ischemia persists and BP remains elevated. Titrate to effect) and/or
Nitroprusside
start 0.1–5.0 μg/kg per min IV

* Base management after this point on invasive hemodynamic monitoring if possible.
† Fluid bolus of 250–500 mL normal saline should be tried. If no response, consider sympathomimetics.
‡ Move to *dopamine* and stop *norepinephrine* when BP improves.
§ Add *dopamine* (and avoid *dobutamine*) if systolic BP drops below 100 mm Hg.

Fig. 8. Algorithm for hypotension, shock, and acute pulmonary edema. (JAMA 268[16]: 2227.)

Algorithm for Initial Evaluation of Suspected Stroke

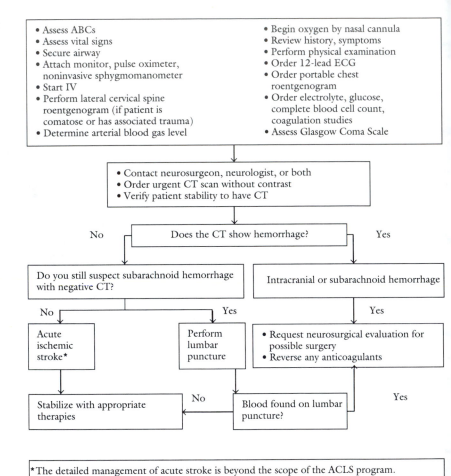

- Assess ABCs
- Assess vital signs
- Secure airway
- Attach monitor, pulse oximeter, noninvasive sphygmomanometer
- Start IV
- Perform lateral cervical spine roentgenogram (if patient is comatose or has associated trauma)
- Determine arterial blood gas level

- Begin oxygen by nasal cannula
- Review history, symptoms
- Perform physical examination
- Order 12-lead ECG
- Order portable chest roentgenogram
- Order electrolyte, glucose, complete blood cell count, coagulation studies
- Assess Glasgow Coma Scale

- Contact neurosurgeon, neurologist, or both
- Order urgent CT scan without contrast
- Verify patient stability to have CT

No — Does the CT show hemorrhage? — Yes

Do you still suspect subarachnoid hemorrhage with negative CT?

Intracranial or subarachnoid hemorrhage

No — Yes

Yes

Acute ischemic stroke*

Perform lumbar puncture

- Request neurosurgical evaluation for possible surgery
- Reverse any anticoagulants

Stabilize with appropriate therapies

No — Blood found on lumbar puncture? — Yes

*The detailed management of acute stroke is beyond the scope of the ACLS program. Management of cardiovascular emergencies in stroke victims is similar to the management in other patients. Never forget, however, that acute stroke can coexist with acute cardiovascular problems.

Fig. 10. Algorithm for initial evaluation of suspected stroke. (JAMA 268[16]:2243.)

Algorithm for Treatment of Hypothermia

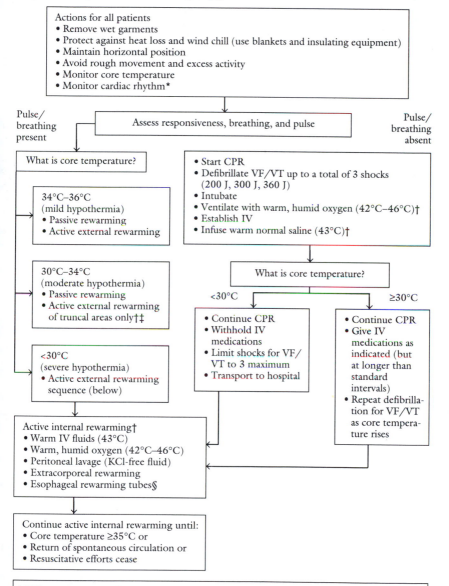

Actions for all patients
- Remove wet garments
- Protect against heat loss and wind chill (use blankets and insulating equipment)
- Maintain horizontal position
- Avoid rough movement and excess activity
- Monitor core temperature
- Monitor cardiac rhythm*

Pulse/breathing present

Assess responsiveness, breathing, and pulse

Pulse/breathing absent

What is core temperature?

34°C–36°C
(mild hypothermia)
- Passive rewarming
- Active external rewarming

- Start CPR
- Defibrillate VF/VT up to a total of 3 shocks (200 J, 300 J, 360 J)
- Intubate
- Ventilate with warm, humid oxygen (42°C–46°C)†
- Establish IV
- Infuse warm normal saline (43°C)†

30°C–34°C
(moderate hypothermia)
- Passive rewarming
- Active external rewarming of truncal areas only†‡

What is core temperature?

<30°C

≥30°C

<30°C
(severe hypothermia)
- Active external rewarming sequence (below)

- Continue CPR
- Withhold IV medications
- Limit shocks for VF/VT to 3 maximum
- Transport to hospital

- Continue CPR
- Give IV medications as indicated (but at longer than standard intervals)
- Repeat defibrillation for VF/VT as core temperature rises

Active internal rewarming†
- Warm IV fluids (43°C)
- Warm, humid oxygen (42°C–46°C)
- Peritoneal lavage (KCl-free fluid)
- Extracorporeal rewarming
- Esophageal rewarming tubes§

Continue active internal rewarming until:
- Core temperature ≥35°C or
- Return of spontaneous circulation or
- Resuscitative efforts cease

* This may require needle electrodes through the skin.
† Many experts think these interventions should be done only in-hospital though practices vary.
‡ Methods include electric or charcoal warming devices, hot water bottles, heating pads, radiant heat sources, and warming beds.
§ Esophageal rewarming tubes are widely used internationally and should become available in the United States.

Fig. 11. Algorithm for treatment of hypothermia. (JAMA 268[16]:2245.)

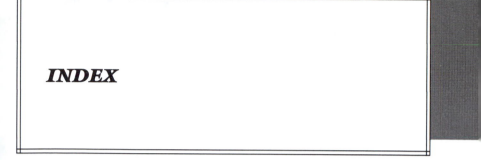

INDEX

A

Aarane, action/dosage/side effects of, 96
Absorption, gastrointestinal secretions
    related to, 188–90
Acebutolol, 15, 18
Acetaminophen poisoning, 231–32
Acid-base balance
    abnormalities in, 104
    compensation vs. correction of,
        67
    disorders, signs/symptoms of, 68
Acidosis
    compensation for, 69
    metabolic, causes of, 67
    respiratory, causes of, 66
ACLS guidelines
    algorithm for pulseless electrical
        activity, 22
    algorithm for ventricular fibrillation and
        pulseless ventricular tachycardia, 21
    aystole treatment algorithm, 23
    tachycardia algorithm, 24
    universal algorithm for adult emergency
        cardiac care, 20
Acute confusion
    possible reversible causes of, 6
    symptoms of, 5
Acute disseminated intravascular coagula-
    tion (DIC), 212
Acute gastrointestinal bleeding, diagnostic
    findings for, 195
Acute myocardial infarction
    nursing care plan for patient with,
        276–83
    patient/family education following, 42
Acute pancreatitis
    assessment of, 196
    causes of, 195
    complications of, 197
    management of, 197
    nursing care plan for, 330–33
Acute renal failure (ARF). *See also* Renal
        failure
    causes of, 110
    diagnosis of, 110
    general categories of, 109
    nursing care plan for patient with
        intrarenal, 301–2
        postrenal, 303–4
        prerenal azotemia, 299–300
    treatment for, comparison of hemo-

dialysis and peritoneal dialysis
    in, 112
Acute respiratory distress syndrome
    (ARDS)
    clinical assessment of, 91
    nursing care plan for patient with,
        284–89
Acute transmural myocardial infarctions,
    electrocardiogram changes for, 38
Acute tubular necrosis, differentiation of
    decreased renal perfusion from, 111
Adenosine, pharmacokinetics of, 17
Adrenal crisis
    nursing care plan for patient in, 334–35
    signs/symptoms of, 205
Aging, cognitive changes with, 6
AIDS
    case definition for, 241
    clinical manifestations of, 243–45
    epidemiology of, 240
    nursing care plan for patient with,
        342–45
    phases of, 242
Airway placement, 71
Albuterol, action/dosage/side effects of, 93
Alfentanil, in anesthetic options, 249
ALG. *See* Antilymphocyte globulin (ALG)
Alkalosis
    causes of, 66
    compensation for, 69
AlkaSeltzer poisoning, 234
ALS. *See* Antilymphocyte serum (ALS)
Alupent, action/dosage/side effects of, 93
Amikacin, dosage of, in renal failure, 113
Aminoglycosides
    dosage of, in renal failure, 113
    effects of nondepolarizing muscle relax-
        ants increased by, 253
Aminophylline, halothane and, cardiac
    dysrhythmias associated with, 252
Amiodarone, 15
    pharmacokinetics of, 17
Amiodipine, comparison of, 18
Amitriptyline poisoning, 228
Amoxapine poisoning, 228
Amoxicillin, dosage of, in renal failure,
    114
Amphetamine poisoning, 223–24
Ampicillin, dosage of, in renal failure, 114
Analgesia, epidural, side effects from, man-
        agement of, 256